Renew Your Life:
Improved Digestion and Detoxification

By Brenda Watson, N.D., C.T.

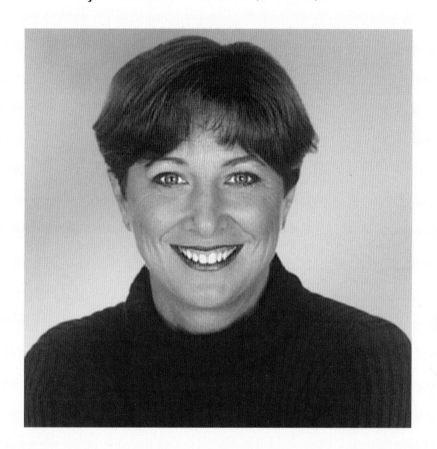

with Susan Stockton, M.A
Foreword by Leonard Smith, M.D.

Renew Your Life:
Improved Digestion and Detoxification

By Brenda Watson, N.D., C.T.
with Susan Stockton, M.A.
Foreword by Leonard Smith, M.D.

Third Printing
Renew Life Press and Information Services
2076 Sunnydale Drive
Clearwater, FL 33765
1-866-450-1784

Acknowledgements

The gratitude and thanks I feel for all the teachers in my life goes beyond the list here. The thousands of clients with whom I have worked and the people to whom I've lectured across the country were the inspiration to create this book. The need for simplification of the digestion and detoxification processes is the primary motivation for this book.

I thank Susan Stockton for her help and guidance in creating this book. Her persistence in keeping me focused on this project is the reason we have this finished book. Her vast knowledge of natural healing and writing contributed greatly to the shaping of this book.

Thank you, Leonard Smith M.D., for your contribution of information and unique perspectives, traditional as well as holistic. Also, your constant optimism and love helped make this an easier process.

To the family of ReNew Life and Advanced Naturals, your love and constant support of me and the endeavors of the company makes me very grateful and proud. I could not have asked for a better support group during this process. A special thanks to Kathi Murray for her knowledge and creativity in the design of this book.

Much thanks and appreciation to Ed Gazsi for his creativity and talent in drawing many of the illustrations in the book.

A special thanks to my children (Joy and Travis) who have been instrumental in this process of creating a support system for me.

Most of all, I wish to acknowledge my husband, Stan Watson, for his constant support and participation in the writing and editing of this book. His endless support has been one of the main reasons for my success in this field. He has been unselfish in creating the space for me to travel endlessly with this message.

Brenda Watson, N.D., C.T.
Clearwater, FL
2002

Preface

After many years of lecturing across the country to thousands of people about the digestive system and the detoxification process, I began to think about writing this book. At each lecture I knew the explanation of the digestive process needed to be simplified and made 'real' to people through the use of pictures and charts. Such visual aids make the information easier to understand.

My personal struggle with poor health made me aware that detoxification is important, whether you're trying to regain health (as I was) or maintain it. In either case, detoxifying the body (ridding it of poisons) and improving the digestive process are necessary.

I regained my health many years ago largely through colon hydrotherapy and herbal supplementation. At that time, such therapeutic practices as fasting and colonics were considered 'strange' by most people. The natural healing philosophy has become more accepted during the last two decades, and so too have such therapies. The holistic approach to healing is being increasingly viewed as 'scientific' with the accreditation of a growing number of naturopathic colleges. The development and use of specialized laboratory tests to aid physicians in diagnosing such digestive disorders as dysbiosis has also made natural healing philosophy and practices more acceptable.

During my career, I have worked in – and developed my own – clinics that specialize in digestion and detoxification. In doing so, I have seen many people regain their health and better maintain it through the application of natural healing principles. This has inspired me and given rise to a passion for my work – a passion that remains to this day, which has resulted in a renewed commitment to health education.

I am confident that the information contained in this book will enable you, the reader, to better understand the digestive system and its function. Knowledge is power. The information in *Renew Your Life* will empower you to make the best health choices and quite literally renew your life! It has been said that "the digestive system is like the roots of a tree; when the roots are diseased, the whole tree is affected." Nutrition, digestion, absorption, bacterial balance and intestinal permeability all play interdependent functions in the health of the gastrointestinal tract and the health of the whole body. All are presented in this book.

Brenda Watson, N.D., C.T.
(Colon Therapist)

P.S. In reading through this book, you'll note that at times I use the word 'I,' and at other times, I use the word 'we.' 'I' is used when the opinion expressed or experience described is my own. When 'we' is used, that opinion/experience is one that is shared by my co-author, Susan Stockton.

Foreword

As a board certified surgeon I have, during the last 25 years, operated on thousands of people with digestive disorders. By the time these patients arrive at my office they are often well into a chronic disease state. I have often asked myself, "What could this person have done to avoid this surgery?" In many cases, the answer is that these operations could have been prevented with diet and lifestyle modifications. Going a step further, I am convinced that the majority of all diseases could be avoided or modified with a proper understanding of nutrition, digestion, elimination and stress modification.

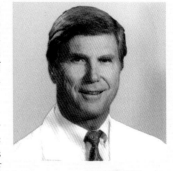

These 'digestive care' concepts are not new: Taking the time to eat clean food, chewing thoroughly, eating probiotics (good bacteria like acidophilus and bifidiobacteria), taking digestive enzymes, eating raw foods, and consuming optimum amounts of fiber and essential fatty acids are basic health guidelines that have been known and practiced worldwide for thousands of years. Our modern society has diluted these key digestive concepts with advertisements for 'fast food,' fad diets and medical advice that promotes a variety of pills in an attempt to control digestive problems rather than address the causes. Proper digestion, elimination and detoxification are the cornerstones of vibrant health. The skyrocketing incidence of chronic illnesses in the U.S.A. will continue until we embrace and promote these digestive care concepts.

The medical literature is replete with clinical data to support the various facets of digestive care and detoxification. Many of the books on the subject are as difficult to read as the clinical studies. Brenda Watson has done an excellent job defining and clarifying the most important digestive care principles. This book is complete in its attention to data but simple in the delivery of the information. Both medical practitioners and all others interested in digestive care and detoxification will find this book to be most helpful in increasing their understanding in this area.

Leonard Smith, M.D.
Gainesville, Florida, 2002

Table of Contents

CHAPTER 10
Dietary Guidelines for Health Maintenance . .121

CHAPTER 11
Managing Digestive Conditions 137

CHAPTER 12
Children 155

Appendix 168

Digestive Care™

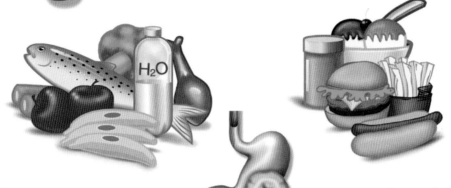
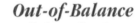

In-Balance

A healthy digestive tract has a semi-permeable mucosal lining that helps prevent undigested food and toxins from entering the bloodstream. Fully digested nutrients and liquids may pass through to nourish the body.

Out-of-Balance

An out-of-balance digestive tract can have a porous mucosal lining. Undigested foods and toxins can pass through to enter the bloodstream.

Leaky Gut

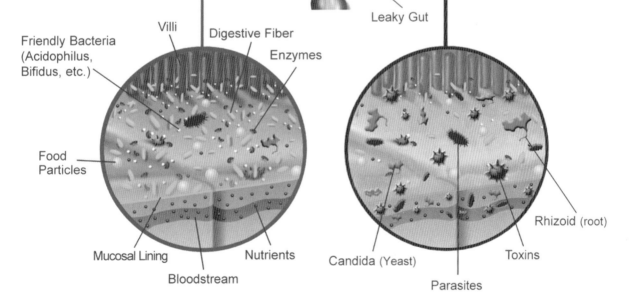

Villi

Friendly Bacteria
(Acidophilus,
Bifidus, etc.)

Digestive Fiber

Enzymes

Food
Particles

Mucosal Lining

Bloodstream

Nutrients

Candida (Yeast)

Parasites

Toxins

Rhizoid (root)

Renew Your Life
Introduction

What is more valuable to you than good health? Your family? Your faith in a higher power? A hefty bank balance? A good movie? A new car? Well, guess what? You can't enjoy any of them if you have poor health. If you are sick, exhausted, or in pain, you will simply not have the time or energy to enjoy all the things that life has to offer. You will spend all your time, money and energy trying to deal with your poor health, rather than creating a better life for yourself, your family, your community and maybe even the rest of us.

So, you may ask, "What can I do about my poor health?" Well, you can do a great deal. With very few exceptions, we do not suddenly wake up one day with poor health. I'll let you in on a secret: We create our own poor health. How do we do that? Well, we eat too much, drink too much, exercise too little and generally abuse our bodies during a long period of time. We live stressful lives in stressful cities that are full of too many people. We breathe toxic air, drink polluted water and generally pass bacteria and viruses around so often that it is amazing we survive at all. The fact that we do survive for decades in relatively good health is, in part, a testament to the strength of our digestive systems. That's right, I said our 'digestive systems.' It is not natural to drink chlorinated water or homogenized milk; nor are we naturally designed to eat food that has been irradiated, filled with preservatives or coated with pesticides, but that's what we do every day. Through it all, our digestive systems function for years to break down foods and liquids into the few nutrients that are available. Our digestive systems don't stop there. They also help to filter and eliminate toxins, parasites, fungi, bacteria and viruses. It has long been known that health comes from the body's ability to digest nutrients and eliminate waste. The digestive system is responsible for assuring that you:

- Digest foods completely
- Eliminate wastes naturally

The more efficiently your body performs these functions, the healthier you are likely to be.

Do you remember the saying, 'You are what you eat?' There is certainly truth in it. More accurately however, you are what you digest (break down), absorb (take into the bloodstream) and assimilate (take into the cells). The problem is that not all the food we consume is properly utilized. Even assuming that we eat the highest quality food available (most of us do not), we cannot achieve optimal health unless our digestive systems are functioning at their peak.

Aging, poor food quality, faulty preparation methods, external toxins or parasites can lead to a premature decline of our digestive systems and long term chronic disease. These diseases can include arthritis, diabetes, fibromyalgia, chronic fatigue, Alzheimer's, irritable bowel syndrome and many others. When our digestive systems do not function correctly, we are not able to reap the full benefit of the food we eat, regardless of how nutrient-dense it may be. Proper digestion is only half the story: To achieve optimal health, our bodies or systems must also eliminate wastes and toxins quickly and efficiently.

Proper elimination of toxins is particularly problematic. In today's world, more than ever, we are exposed to a wide variety of toxins: They're in our air, food and water, in the workplace and at home. We even generate toxins within our own bodies. These toxins produce irritation and inflammation, adding to the burden of the digestive system. When the digestive system becomes overwhelmed, it is no longer able to adequately perform detoxification functions. This is a condition called 'toxic overload.'

Now, before you quit your stressful job, obtain a divorce, move to the forest and live in a cave, you may want to think about what you can do to keep your digestive system healthy. Unfortunately, you can't do much about your age, but you can help your digestive system function at optimal levels by giving your body the proper nutrients and by keeping the digestive system clean and well maintained. Just as you would never run your car engine for 75 years without cleaning it and changing the oil, you cannot run your digestive system forever without proper cleansing and detoxification. Cleansing and detoxification are the natural processes used by the body to rid it of the toxins found in the environment (exotoxins), as well as those created by the body internally (endotoxins). For thousands of years, people have used detoxification and cleansing methods to maintain and restore good health. Cleansing and detoxification programs have increased in popularity in recent years. However, many of the programs are too complicated to follow and maintain. Today's busy lifestyles call for new approaches to cleansing and detoxification – approaches that are safe, effective and simple. As a colon therapist for the last decade, it has been my pleasure to work with thousands of people with digestive disorders and to see many of them restore and renew their health by first improving the ability of their digestive systems to function properly. I have helped thousands of women and men develop cleansing and detoxification programs that fit their lifestyles and unique clinical conditions.

This book has three basic sections. The first section (chapter 1) will provide you with an overview of how a healthy digestive system should function. The second section (chapters 2-5) is full of information on digestive dysfunctions and their causes. The final section

(chapter 6-12) is about achieving optimal digestion. In this section, you will learn what steps you can take to help restore your digestive system to its maximum potential. In the pages that follow, you will learn what happens to your food from the time it enters the mouth until it leaves the body. Furthermore, you will learn what can go wrong in the process and why. AND – most importantly – you'll learn how to avoid, as well as correct and reverse, problems with digestion and elimination. This book will provide you with the knowledge and information you need to achieve optimal and vibrant health; but as in all things in life, you must take the first step.

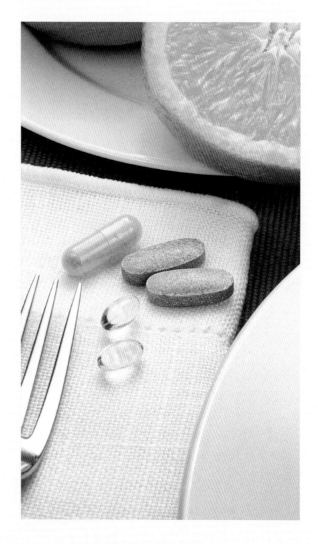

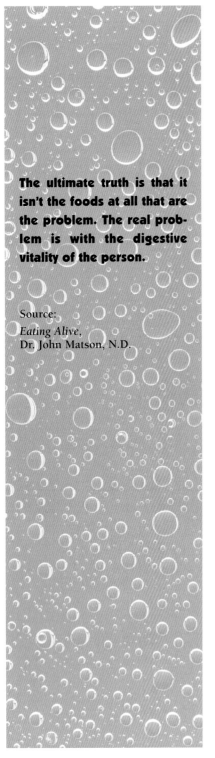

CHAPTER 1

THE HEALTHY digestive SYSTEM

It is estimated that as much as 40% of the population suffer from some form of digestive stress. If you are reading this book, you probably are within this group. You may be unconcerned with the details of the digestive process or just want to know how to be or become healthy. If that is your goal, then the journey to achieving that goal begins with a clear understanding of a healthy digestive system.

WHAT IS DIGESTION?

Digestion encompasses the chemical and motor (physical motion) activities that separate food into its most basic components so that they can be absorbed through the lining of the small intestine. Digestion is the process of converting food into chemical substances that can be absorbed and assimilated. It begins in the mouth and ends in the **large intestine** or **colon**.

What Does the Digestive System Do?

The digestive system has two broad functions: The first and best known is the digestion and absorption of food. The second function is the excretion of wastes. Both of these occur primarily in the small and large intestines; hence the phrase by Gloria Gilbère, ND (Naturopathic Doctor), "The road to health is paved with good intestines."

What Organs Make Up the Digestive System?

The digestive tract is a tube (about 30 feet long) that begins with the mouth and ends with the anus. The digestive system (or gastrointestinal tract) is made up of the mouth, esophagus, stomach, small intestine, large intestine and anus. Along this tube are accessory organs like the teeth, tongue, salivary glands, gallbladder, liver and pancreas.

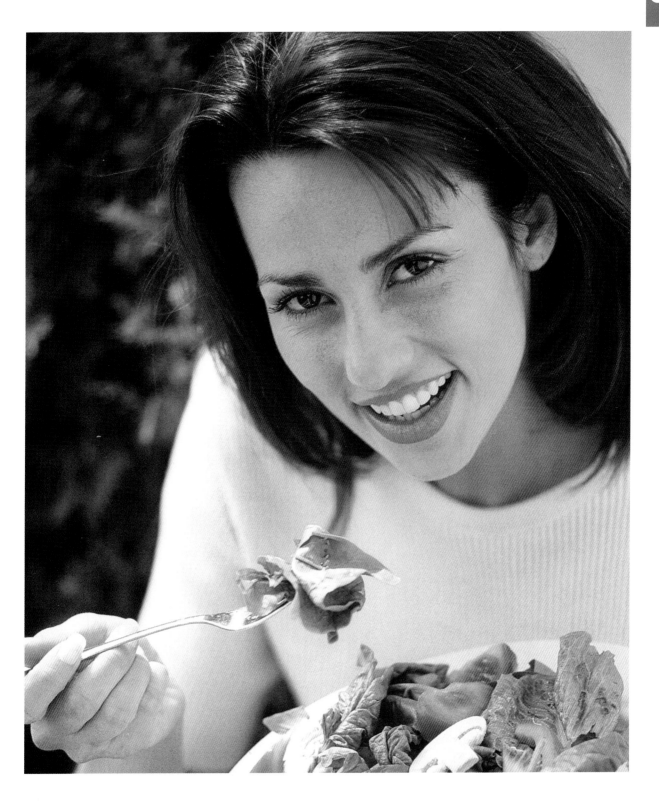

What Are the Functions of the Digestive System?

The digestive tract has three primary functions:

- **Motor** – assisting food movement
- **Secretory** – preparing food for absorption by producing digestive enzymes
- **Absorptive** – breaking food down and converting it into substances that can be absorbed through digestion

THE DIGESTIVE PROCESS

Digestion begins in the mouth where the teeth chew food into smaller particles. Then saliva coats and softens those food particles with **enzymes** (**ptyalin** and **amylase**) that break down carbohydrates (starches and sugars). Saliva also contains enzymes, such as **lysozyme**, that attack bacteria and their protein coats directly. This is the body's first line of defense against parasites and foreign invaders. Once chewing is completed (and sometimes even when it is not), food is swallowed and transferred down the **esophagus** to the stomach.

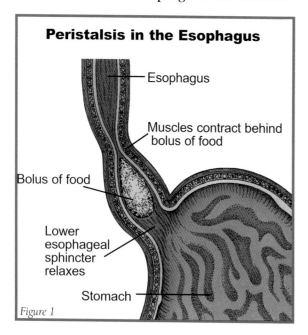

Figure 1

The Esophagus

The esophagus is a 10-inch long muscular tube, lined with mucus-producing cells, which lubricates the food so that it passes through with ease. The esophagus transports food to the stomach through the action of its wave-like muscular contractions (**peristalsis**). It is coated with a protective mucous lining. The muscular valve at the bottom of the esophagus is known as the **lower esophageal sphincter**. This valve remains tightly closed when food is not being eaten so that stomach acid cannot back into the esophagus and cause heartburn. It opens and closes quickly to allow food to pass into the **stomach**.

The Stomach

Many people are surprised to find that very little absorption actually occurs in the stomach. The mucous cells of the stomach can absorb some water, short-chain fatty acids and certain drugs, such as alcohol and aspirin, but the stomach is essentially a holding and mixing tank for food. Its main functions are storage and preliminary digestion. The stomach functions like a big blender, churning and liquefying food. The properly functioning stomach secretes five

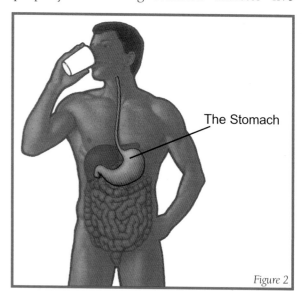

Figure 2

important substances: (1) mucus, (2) **hydrochloric acid** (HCl), (3) a precursor of the protein-digesting enzyme **pepsin**, (4) **gastrin**, a hormone to regulate acid production and (5) gastric **lipase**, which assists in the digestion of fat.

A mucous lining coats the cells of the stomach to protect them from the HCl and enzymes that must be present for proper digestion. This alkaline mucous lining can be damaged by dehydration, over-consumption of food or aspirin, or by the bacterium **Helicobacter pylori** (H. pylori). This damage can often lead to **gastritis** (irritation of the stomach lining) or to a stomach ulcer.

> Contrary to popular belief, many Americans who suffer from heartburn produce too little Hydrocloric Acid (HCl), not too much. Without enough HCl, you may not be able to sufficiently break down proteins. This can lead to bloating, gas and heartburn. Low HCl production can also result in problems with bacterial infections or parasites.

Hydrochloric acid (HCl) is produced by **parietal** cells (tiny pumps) in the lining of the stomach. This acid is needed to ensure the proper functioning of the stomach. HCl has two primary functions: It provides the acidic environment necessary for the enzyme pepsin to break down proteins; and it helps prevent infection by destroying most parasites and bacteria.

At the end of the stomach is the **pyloric sphincter**, which controls the opening between the end of the stomach and the **duodenum**, the first section of the small intestine.

The Duodenum

When food leaves the stomach, it enters the first section of the small intestine known as the duodenum. It is now called **chyme**, a mixture of food, HCl and mucus, which is approximately the consistency of split pea soup. As the duodenum fills, hormones released from the duodenal lining (1) delay gastric emptying, (2) promote bile flow from the liver and gallbladder and (3) promote secretion of water, **bicarbonate** and potent digestive enzymes from the pancreas. The surface of the duodenum is smooth for the first few inches, but quickly changes to a surface with many folds and small finger-like projections called **villi** or **microvilli** (*very* small projections). These projections serve to increase the surface area and absorption capabilities of the duodenum. Properly functioning accessory organs (liver, gallbladder and pancreas) are crucial during this first stage of digestion.

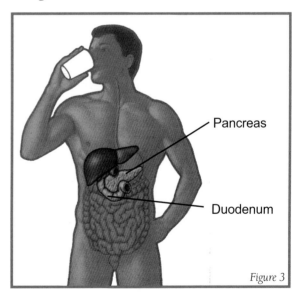

Pancreas

Duodenum

Figure 3

The Pancreas

The **pancreas** is a 6-inch long accessory organ that has three main functions important to digestion:

1. Neutralizes stomach acid
2. Regulates blood sugar levels
3. Produces digestive enzymes

Digestive enzymes digest proteins, carbohydrates and fats. The **proteolytic** (protein-digesting pancreatic) enzymes are secreted in an inactive form and are only activated once they reach the duodenum. The other pancreatic enzymes are secreted in an active form but require **ions** (electrically charged molecules) or bile to be present for optimal activity. Bicarbonates are alkaline and serve to neutralize stomach acid and activate digestive enzymes. These secretions (pancreatic enzymes and bicarbonates) are delivered directly into the duodenum, the upper portion of the small intestine. The pancreas also secretes hormones, which help manage blood sugar levels, directly into the bloodstream. These hormones are **insulin** (sugar lowering) and **glucagon** (sugar raising).

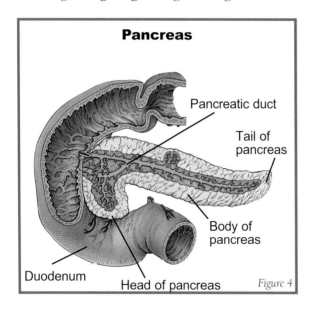

Pancreas

Pancreatic duct

Tail of pancreas

Body of pancreas

Duodenum

Head of pancreas

Figure 4

The Liver and Gallbladder
The **liver** has several important functions, many of which are related to digestion. It produces about half the body's **cholesterol** (the rest comes from food). About 80% of the cholesterol produced by the liver is used to make **bile**. Bile is composed of bile salts, hormones and toxins. It acts to emulsify and distribute fat, cholesterol and fat-soluble vitamins throughout the intestines. Bile

The Pancreas Produces
Bicarbonate – neutralizes stomach acid
Enzymes – digest carbohydrates, fats and protein
Insulin – regulates blood sugar levels

is an alkaline substance that neutralizes stomach acid. Between meals, it is stored in the gallbladder, a pear-shaped organ located just below the liver. When food (chyme) enters the duodenum, a signal is sent to the gallbladder to contract, thereby releasing bile into the **small intestine**.

The Small Intestine
Ninety percent of all nutrients are absorbed in the small intestine, the body's major digestive organ. The small intestine resembles a coiled hose and is approximately 20 feet long. It is here that most food is completely digested and absorbed. The small intestine contains cells that serve many functions: Some produce mucus, some make enzymes, some absorb nutrients and others are capable of killing bacteria. The cells are arranged in folds upon folds, which force the chyme to move slower so it can be broken down completely and absorbed. These folds also increase the surface area of the **mucosa**, the thin mucous membrane lining the walls of the small intestine.

The small intestine consists of three sections – the **duodenum**, the **jejunum** and the **ileum**. The duodenum (first foot of the small intestine) connects to the jejunum, which in turn connects to the ileum. The duodenum primarily absorbs minerals. The jejunum absorbs water-soluble vitamins, carbohydrates and proteins. The ileum absorbs fat-soluble vitamins, fat, cholesterol and bile salts. The walls of the small intestine secrete alkaline digestive enzymes, which continue the separation of foods – proteins into amino acids, fats into fatty acids and glycerin and carbohydrates into simple sugars.

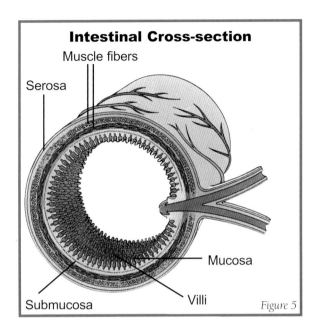

Intestinal Cross-section

Muscle fibers

Serosa

Mucosa

Villi

Submucosa

Figure 5

two-thirds of stool is water, undigested fiber and food products; one-third is living and dead bacteria (bacteria naturally live in the colon). The lowest portion of the descending colon is the **sigmoid**. The sigmoid colon empties into the rectum. In this area, three valves regulate the fecal matter. They are called the **valves of Houston**. This area is normally empty unless defecation is in process.

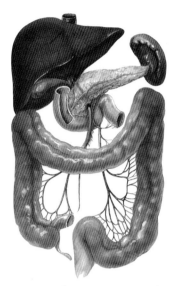

Final stages of digestion occur in the colon with the absorption of water and nutrients not absorbed by the small intestine. The liquid and nutrients are absorbed through the intestinal wall, collected by the blood vessels in the wall lining and carried to the liver through the portal vein for filtration.

The Colon or Large Intestine

The last organ through which food residue passes is the colon or large intestine. The three major segments are the **ascending** (right side of body), **transverse** (connects right to left side) and **descending** (left side). Chyme enters the ascending colon through the **ileocecal valve** (ICV), a one-way valve that connects the small and large intestines and regulates the flow of chyme entering the large intestines. The ICV is designed to let waste pass into the colon and prevent it from backing into the small intestine. When chyme passes through the ICV, then into the very lowest portion of the ascending colon, known as the **cecum**, it is still in a liquid state. The cecum is the first section of the five feet of colon. Food waste travels up the ascending colon (through rhythmic waves of contraction or peristalsis), across the transverse and down the descending portion of the organ. As it moves across the transverse colon, liquid is extracted. It is the job of the colon to absorb water and nutrients from the chyme and to form feces. The fecal matter is in a semi-solid state, gradually becoming firmer, as it approaches the descending colon. About

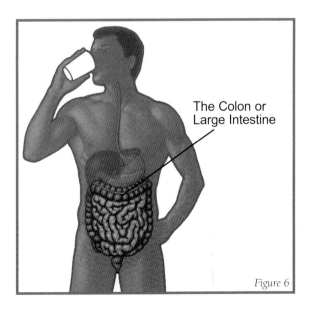

The Colon or Large Intestine

Figure 6

The large intestine also:

1. Secretes bicarbonate to neutralize acid end products
2. Stores waste products, bacteria and intestinal gas
3. Excretes poisons and waste products from the body

The **rectum** is the chamber at the end of the large intestine. Fecal matter passes into the rectum, creating the urge to defecate. The **anus** is the opening at the far end of the digestive tract. The anus allows fecal matter to pass out of the body. The anal sphincters keep the anus closed.

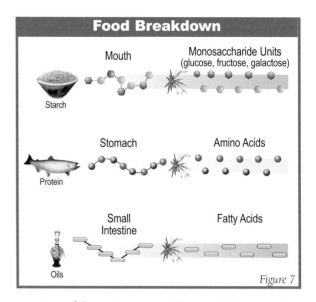

Figure 7

The Mucous Membrane

The walls of both the small and large intestines consist of four layers. The innermost layer of the small intestine is called the mucosa. The mucosa has two very important functions: First, it is designed to allow nutrients of the proper size to pass through it and into the bloodstream. Second, the mucosa blocks the passage of undigested food particles, parasites, bacteria and toxins into the bloodstream. Therefore, the mucosa or mucosal lining is a vital part of the body's immune system because it limits the volume of potential invaders. The mucosa is lined with villi and microvilli. The villi are moving absorptive cells that 'suck up' small particles of digested food. On each of the villi are thousands of tiny projections of the membrane of the cell called microvilli. These little brush-like fuzzy structures (called the '**brush border**') further amplify the surface area of the small intestines. **Stretched end to end with all its folds, the small intestine has the approximate surface area of a tennis court.**

On the surface of this mucosal lining is a thick mucous layer whose surface (the **glycocalyx**) is highly viscous (slippery). Much of the mucus

consists of the amino sugar **N-acetyl-glucosamine** (NAG). The body makes NAG from the amino acid **L-glutamine**. L-glutamine exists in virtually all cells, and it is one of the most prevalent amino acids in the body. Humans must have L-glutamine in order to produce NAG and have a healthy mucosal lining. The mucosal lining in a healthy person sheds and then is rebuilt every three to five days. Studies have shown that individuals suffering from any inflammatory bowel disease shed this mucosal layer at a much higher rate. This may be due to an inability to convert L-glutamine into NAG.

THE DIGESTIVE ENVIRONMENT

It is difficult to fully understand the digestive system without realizing the importance of the bacteria and microbes that live in the intestinal tract. A newborn baby has essentially no digestive bacteria. Within a few hours, the bacteria and microbes begin to colonize the digestive tract. It has been observed that breast-fed babies develop a larger colony of friendly strains of **bifidobacteria** than those who are bottle-fed. Ideally, pregnant women should supplement with the friendly bacteria

Healthy Digestive Tract

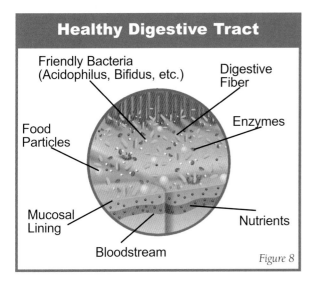

Friendly Bacteria
(Acidophilus, Bifidus, etc.)

Digestive
Fiber

Food
Particles

Enzymes

Mucosal
Lining

Nutrients

Bloodstream

Figure 8

These microbes exist throughout the digestive system from the mouth to the anus, but most of the bacteria live in the large intestine. (The stomach is so acidic that almost no bacteria can live there.) The large intestine can contain as many as four pounds of these microbial creatures at any one time. Approximately 500 different species of microbes live in the digestive system, but only 30 to 40 species constitute 99% of the microbes in the intestinal tract. In terms of how these microbes affect the body, they can be placed into one of three categories:

1. Good (or symbiotic)
2. Neutral
3. Bad

In a healthy person, there is a ratio of approximately 80–85% combined good and neutral bacteria to 15–20% bad. In many people today, this ratio is reversed. Faulty digestion can contribute to this imbalance.

The good bacteria are sometimes called '**flora**' or '**probiotics**.' These good bacteria are beneficial because they:

1. Produce enzymes that help digest foods (e.g., lactase enzyme digests milk)
2. Produce the vitamins B, A and K
3. Produce **lactic acid**, which helps acidify the colon
4. Crowd bad bacteria and keep them from becoming too numerous
5. Produce organic acids that may help with fecal elimination by peristalsis
6. Produce short-chain fatty acids (**butyric acid**), which supply energy to intestinal cells

The two most important types of good bacteria are **Lactobacillus** and **Bifidobacteria**.

known as Lactobacillus (L.) acidophilus, and bifidobacteria during the third trimester of pregnancy. Friendly bacteria (also known as probiotics, discussed in chapter 8) are important for babies at the time of birth. L. acidophilus in the vagina inoculates the newborn as he/she passes through the birth canal, and it provides protection from other bacteria, as well as assisting with digestion and with the production of vitamins. The bifidobacteria ingested by the mother is concentrated in the breast milk and is passed on intact to the nursing baby. These two events establish the friendly bacteria in the newborn and greatly decrease the possibility of serious infections that can occur during infancy. The mother can provide friendly bacteria for her baby by ingesting a supplement containing L. acidophilus and bifidobacteria, or by eating yogurt or kefir with live cultures of these bacteria. It may be best to do both, since it is necessary to provide ample amounts of the probiotics on a regular basis.

As adults, our digestive systems contain about 100 trillion bacteria, fungi and microbes. You actually have more bacteria in your gastrointestinal tract than cells in your body!

Digestive Organs

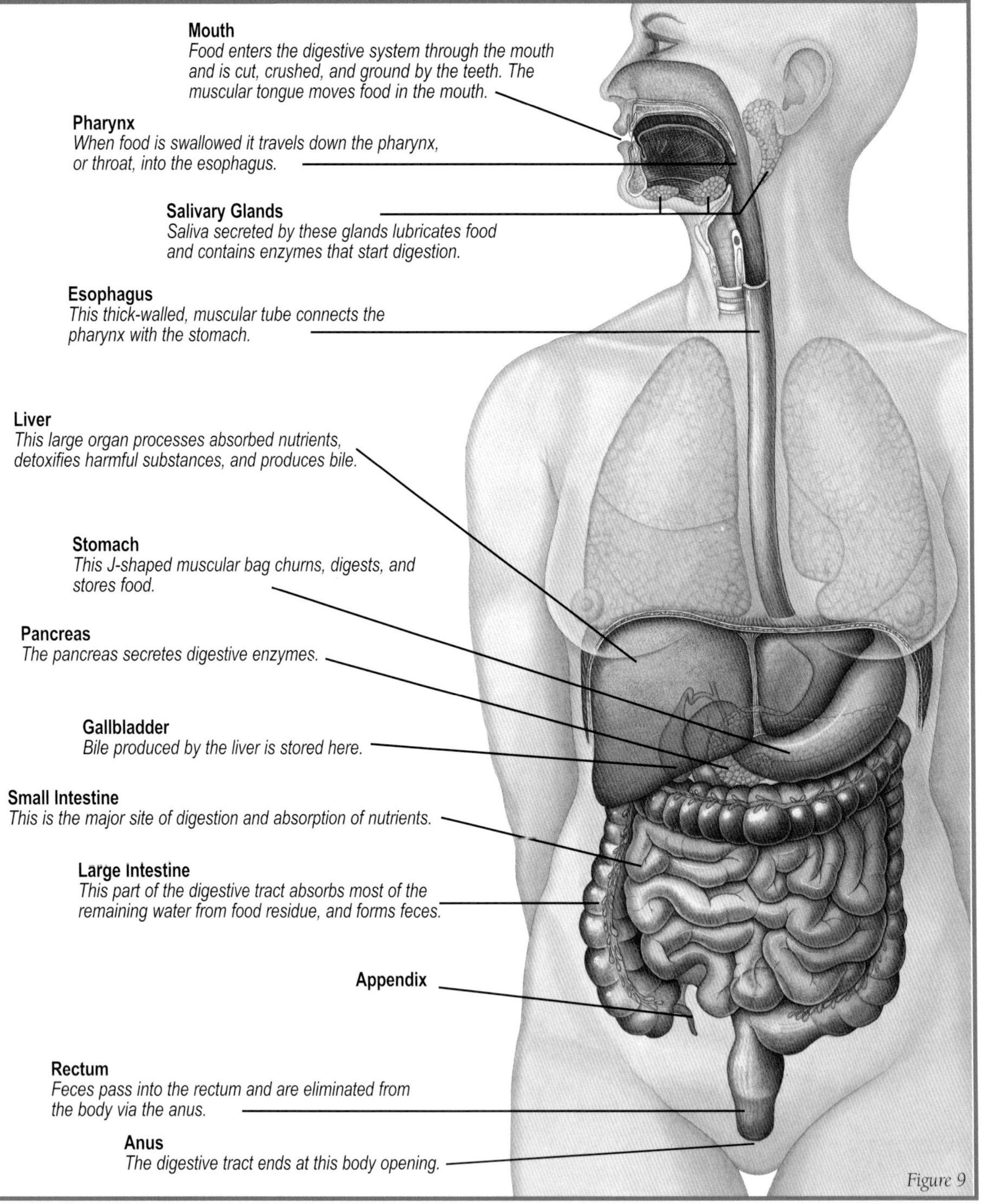

Mouth
Food enters the digestive system through the mouth and is cut, crushed, and ground by the teeth. The muscular tongue moves food in the mouth.

Pharynx
When food is swallowed it travels down the pharynx, or throat, into the esophagus.

Salivary Glands
Saliva secreted by these glands lubricates food and contains enzymes that start digestion.

Esophagus
This thick-walled, muscular tube connects the pharynx with the stomach.

Liver
This large organ processes absorbed nutrients, detoxifies harmful substances, and produces bile.

Stomach
This J-shaped muscular bag churns, digests, and stores food.

Pancreas
The pancreas secretes digestive enzymes.

Gallbladder
Bile produced by the liver is stored here.

Small Intestine
This is the major site of digestion and absorption of nutrients.

Large Intestine
This part of the digestive tract absorbs most of the remaining water from food residue, and forms feces.

Appendix

Rectum
Feces pass into the rectum and are eliminated from the body via the anus.

Anus
The digestive tract ends at this body opening.

Figure 9

Bad bacteria produce substances that are harmful to the body. They irritate the lining of the intestines (causing gas) and can be absorbed into the bloodstream (causing disease). They cannot always be prevented from entering the body, but if the number of good and neutral bacteria stays high, then, theoretically, the bad bacteria will be kept to a minimum. Examples of bad bacteria are **salmonella** and **H. pylori**, the bacterium associated with ulcers.

The neutral bacteria are the most prevalent bacteria in the digestive tract. Neutral microbes have neither a positive nor negative impact.

The levels of these three types of organisms remain relatively constant throughout childhood and mid to late adult years. As we age, the levels of bad bacteria often increase, and the good bacteria decrease.

THE SIGNS OF GOOD DIGESTION AND ELIMINATION

At minimum, one should have one good bowel movement per day, but two to three are ideal. A 'good' bowel movement is one that is walnut brown in color, with a consistency similar to toothpaste, about the length of a banana. The stool should be free of odor, leave the body easily, settle in the toilet water and gently submerge. The **transit time** for food – the elapsed time it takes for a meal to enter the mouth and then exit the rectum – should ideally be less than 24 hours. Transit time is related to exercise and the consumption of fiber and water.

> **When transit time slows, putrefied material stays in the colon longer, and toxins can enter the bloodstream through the intestinal wall.**

THE SEVEN CHANNELS OF ELIMINATION

The seven channels of elimination are:

- Colon
- Lungs
- Liver
- Skin
- Kidneys
- Blood
- Lymph

The first 5 of these channels (column 1) are all organs. The processes of the colon have been explained in this chapter. The liver, the body's primary filtering organ, will be presented in chapter 5. The blood that flows through the vessels of the **vascular** (blood circulatory) system carries oxygen and nutrients to the cells of the body and removes harmful wastes. Not so familiar to many is the other circulatory system, the **lymphatic system**, through which **lymph** flows.

The Lymph

The **lymphatic system** and the vascular system serve to eliminate poisons from cells. The lymphatic system consists of a network of vessels that extends throughout the body, following the path of the veins. The lymphatic capillaries contain a clear

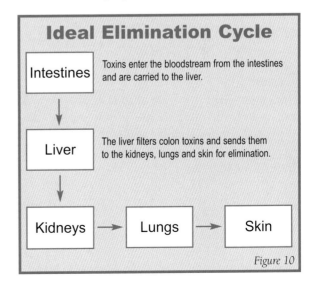

Figure 10

fluid, lymph, which carries **lymphocytes** (immune cells). The lymphatic system is an important part of the immune system. In fact, organs of the immune system are known as 'lymphoid organs.' They include the following:

Bone marrow – where lymphocytes originate

Spleen – a filter for the lymphatic system and a storage site for lymphocytes.

Liver – a major detoxification organ, presented in chapter 5

Lymph nodes – small bean-shaped structures that connect with lymphatic capillaries (They are concentrated in the groin, armpits, neck and abdomen; they filter lymph and produce lymphocytes.)

Thymus gland – home of the **T cells**, which mobilize the body's defense system when it is immune-challenged. See figure 9.

All these lymphoid organs are concerned with the growth, development and deployment of white blood cells (lymphocytes), whose function it is to defend the body against **antigens** (substances the body perceives as foreign and threatening, such as viruses, fungi, bacteria, parasites and pollen).

Kidneys
The **kidneys** are two bean-shaped organs located just under the **diaphragm** in the back. The liver sends water-soluble wastes to the kidneys via the blood where this waste is eliminated through the **bladder**.

Although small enough to fit in the palm of a hand and weighing no more than an orange, the kidneys are considered the 'great purifiers' of the body. Each kidney contains a million individual filter units (globules), and, according to Dr. Henry

> **The gastrointestinal tract has the largest blood supply in the body, taking a third of the blood flow from the heart to get its job done.**
>
> D. Lindsey Berkson,
> *Healthy Digestion the Natural Way*

Bieler, "can filter 1700 quarts of viscous fluid (in which 50 different chemicals are dissolved) in 24 hours."[1] The kidneys determine which of these 50 chemicals are needed by the body, absorb them and filter out the rest. Of the blood filtered by the kidneys, 0.1% becomes urine.[2] The kidneys have the additional function of maintaining water balance.

Lungs
The **lungs**, another secondary elimination organ, expel toxins from the body. One of the most common toxins is **carbon dioxide**. The action of deep breathing helps to move lymph and blood through the body, and with it, toxins. The lungs are lined with mucus and **cilia** (hair-like projections) to help protect against and remove inhaled toxins.

Skin
The **skin** is the body's largest organ. It serves as a protective barrier to prevent toxins from entering the body. Because of its size, the skin "can eliminate more cellular waste than the colon and kidneys combined."[3] It eliminates wastes through its sweat glands and mucous secretions and is considered a secondary elimination organ. The skin protects our inner parts and gauges temperature needs. New skin is made every 24 hours. This skin will be as clean as the blood that flows below it, for the condition of the skin reflects the condition of all that lies beneath it.

There are three layers of skin: the outer, inner and middle layers. The outer skin is the visible layer or 'hide.' The inner skin is called the **mucous membrane**. The middle skin (or **serous membrane**) lines the walls of the lungs, heart, abdomen and pelvic cavities, as well as those of the head and joints.

Notes

[1] Henry G. Bieler, MD, *Food is Your Best Medicine*, Ballantine Books, 1965, p. 45.

[2] Cheryl Townsley, *Cleansing Made Simple*, LFH Publishing, 2001, p. 18.

[3] Ibid., p. 15.

Chapter Summary

Digestion of carbohydrates starts in the mouth through the secretion of the enzymes ptyalin and amylase from the salivary glands. Food travels then through the esophagus into the stomach. The stomach's churning and secretion of digestive juices converts the food to chyme. Pepsin and HCl from the stomach break down protein. Chyme then enters the duodenum, where bicarbonates and digestive enzymes from the pancreas neutralize stomach acid and break down food into its component parts. Bile is secreted from the gallbladder into the duodenum to emulsify fat and decompose it for distribution. Food residue passes next into the small intestine, where 90% of absorption takes place. It then enters the large intestine through the ileocecal valve, traveling up the ascending colon, across the transverse, down the descending colon, through the rectum and out the anus. Liquid and nutrients pass through the wall of the large intestine into the bloodstream, then on to the liver for processing and filtration.

The colon houses three types of bacteria: good, neutral and bad. A balance of approximately 80% good/neutral to 20% bad is desirable for health maintenance. This balance will assist the body in normal elimination of solid waste, a minimum of one daily bowel movement (preferably two to three).

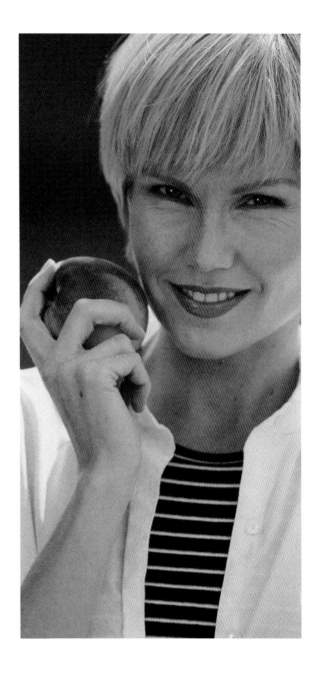

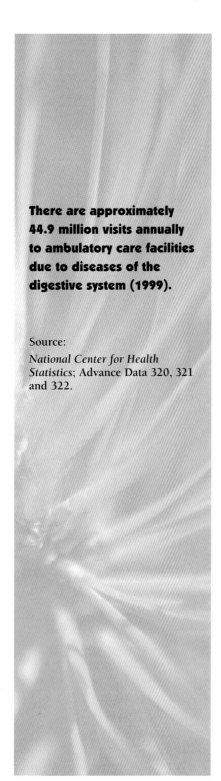

There are approximately 44.9 million visits annually to ambulatory care facilities due to diseases of the digestive system (1999).

Source:
National Center for Health Statistics; Advance Data 320, 321 and 322.

CHAPTER 2

IMPAIRED
digestion

Impaired digestion is the beginning of a process that ends with chronic disease (see figure 1). Throughout, there are many factors that can and do influence the process. Some of the factors are stress, drugs, alcohol, cigarettes, genetics, diet and environmental toxins. The only one not controlled easily in this process is genetics. A closer look at the digestive system reveals the effects of these influences.

Today there are more than sixty million Americans who suffer from digestive disorders, making gastrointestinal complaints the third leading cause of illness in this country. In this chapter, we will examine the causes and clinical implications of impaired digestion. Ultimately, poor digestion will encourage the advancement of age-related illness and autoimmune diseases such as arthritis, fibromyalgia, chronic fatigue, irritable bowel syndrome and more.

Food must be in the proper form for the body to absorb it. For example, carbohydrates must be converted into a form of glucose, and protein into amino acids. If food is not converted properly, it will pass through the system in an undigested form and produce toxins. If these toxins are not promptly eliminated, they can lead to chronic disease. As figure 1 shows, impaired digestion is the beginning of a series of problems that lead ultimately to chronic disease. Many of these problems are part of our daily life:

• Stress
• Processed food consumption
• Inadequate chewing/excess fluid intake with meals
• Improper food combining
• Overeating

When these factors affect our ability to properly digest and process foods, the results can include:

• Lowered production of hydrochloric acid (HCl)

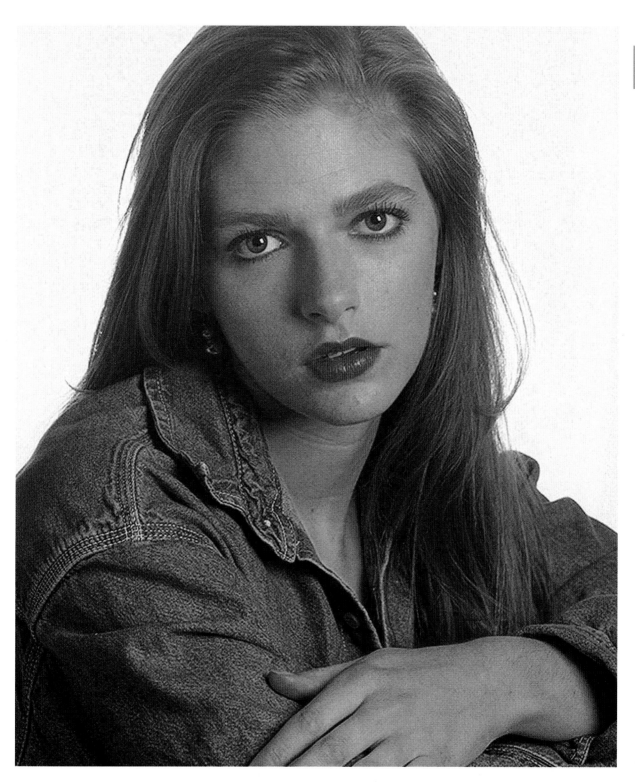

- Pancreatic impairment (reduced enzyme production)
- Imbalanced intestinal pH
- Food sensitivities

The following section explores these factors in more detail.

CAUSES OF POOR DIGESTION

The Role of Stress

There are several reasons why the body fails to digest food properly. A primary cause of poor digestion is stress. All unconscious activity in the body is controlled by the **autonomic nervous system**. The autonomic nervous system controls the digestive system and our reactions to stress. The body is designed to divert energy, blood, enzymes and oxygen away from the digestive organs when stress is experienced. If, for example, we have just eaten breakfast and are late for work, the body will support our mad dash through traffic before it will help digest a meal.

Any type of stress can have an adverse effect on the digestive process, virtually stopping it by lowering pancreatic enzyme production and inhibiting HCl production. Stress can be of a physical, mental or emotional nature.

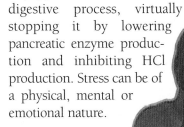

Physical stress is tangible. Infections (even low-grade, subclinical ones), as well as trauma from injuries and surgery, are obvious types of physical stress. Dietary indiscretions (such as

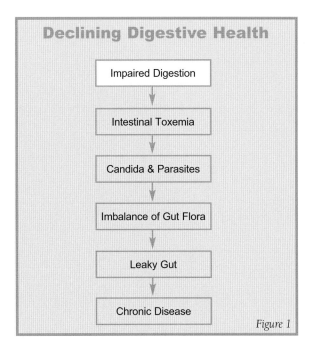

Declining Digestive Health

Impaired Digestion
↓
Intestinal Toxemia
↓
Candida & Parasites
↓
Imbalance of Gut Flora
↓
Leaky Gut
↓
Chronic Disease

Figure 1

high sugar intake) constitute another type of physical stress that can have an adverse effect on the digestive system. Less obvious are more minor physical stressors like noise pollution and minor injuries such as cuts and bruises.

Emotional and **mental stress** – including financial worries, unhappy home life, unfulfilled career aspirations and arguments – all are a strain on the physical body and adversely alter its physiology. Emotional stress causes the body to use its nutritional reserves. Once these nutritional reserves are depleted, digestion becomes impaired, owing to a lack of enzymes needed for the digestive process to function adequately. It's easy to see how any type of emotional or mental stress can become a digestive stress. It is extremely important to cultivate a relaxed state of mind when eating. This ensures unimpaired blood circulation needed for the organs of digestion to work properly.

In today's world, we're literally surrounded by environmental stress in the form of pollution, chemical additives and drugs. Pollutants are primarily man-made chemicals that don't belong in the body but have found their way there through contaminated air and water supplies. A growing number of these will pollute the environment and our bodies, adding more stress to already overburdened systems.

> **There are more than 80,000 toxic chemicals in use today, with 1,200 new ones added annually.**

Chemicals also find their way into the body in the form of additives (approximately 5,000 of them) used to preserve, color, flavor, emulsify and otherwise treat our food. The ingestion of drugs, both prescription and non-prescription, adds more chemical stress. Even a simple visit to the dentist is likely to increase the toxic load on the body. The mercury and other metals in a 'silver' filling can result in oral toxicity, which ultimately causes systemic toxicity. Excessive toxins (chemicals, pollution and drugs) in the body must be processed and removed. This detoxification process uses large amounts of energy, which leaves little energy for proper digestive function. Improper digestion, as noted, can ultimately lead to degenerative and chronic disease.

Processed Food Consumption

Processed foods are those that have been through a commercial refining process, which includes the application of high temperatures. Such processing serves the purpose of increasing shelf life. The down side is that it also destroys some nutrients, creating a situation of imbalance and deficiency.

Refined carbohydrates include all products made with white sugar and flour. During the refining process, these foods are stripped of dozens of essential nutrients, including trace minerals

needed for carbohydrate combustion. A steady diet of refined carbohydrates forces the body to rob itself of the chromium, manganese, cobalt, copper, zinc and magnesium needed to digest the carbohydrates. Once these minerals are depleted, the body is unable to digest carbohydrates properly (processed or natural). Consequently, these partially digested foods will **ferment** into simple sugars and alcohols, providing fuel for yeast and bacteria and leading to indigestion, gas and bloating, which increases the body's toxic load.

Regular intake of refined carbohydrates therefore increases both toxicity and deficiency, creating not only digestive disturbance but ultimately also serious health problems. Refined carbs feed the bad bacteria, irritate digestive organs and reduce the speed and efficiency of digestion.

Fiber is a non-nutritive food component that provides bulk to move food residue through the intestines. It is found naturally in whole grains, fruits and vegetables. When whole grains are milled, the bran and germ portions are discarded, and with them the fiber and many nutrients. Americans typically consume too little fiber and too many refined carbohydrates, and tend to eat inadequate amounts of fruits and vegetables. Lack of fiber results in a slow transit time of food through the digestive tract. According to Michael Murray, ND, the average daily fiber consumption in the U.S. is approximately 20 grams per person[1] (30-40 grams of fiber is needed daily). The result of such a low fiber intake is a transit time of more than 48 hours (more than twice what it should be). Such a slow transit time can result in the absorption of toxins from putrefied fecal material that

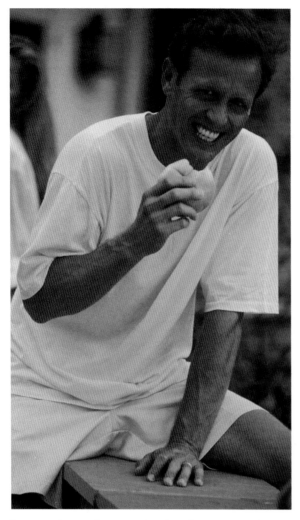

has not been eliminated. The absorption of toxins from within the body's digestive system is a form of self-poisoning or '**autointoxication**,' which can lead to degenerative disease.

The refining process has resulted in fragmentation, not only of grain products but also oil products. Virtually every oil product on supermarket shelves is refined, bleached and deodorized (and not so labeled). During refinement, processed oil products are often exposed to heat, light and oxygen, and are usually extracted with solvents such as hexane (a toxin) to obtain higher yields. Thus much of the quality of the oils is lost in the refinement process.

Many oils are hydrogenated, which increases shelf life at a high cost to consumer health. This process involves the use of extremely high temperatures and super-saturation of the oil with hydrogen, using a nickel catalyst. **Hydrogenation** of oil results in the formation of unnatural '**trans' fatty acids** (TFAs), which constitute 50–60% of the fat content in commonly used 'partially hydrogenated vegetable oils.' Medical research has proven that human consumption of trans fats increases total cholesterol, **LDL** ('bad' cholesterol), and **lipoprotein a**, while decreasing **HDL** ('good' cholesterol), all of which increase the risk of heart disease. Approximately 70% of all the vegetable oils used in food such as crackers, cookies, pastries, cakes, snack chips, imitation cheese, candies and fried foods contain several grams of trans fats.

Inadequate Chewing/Drinking with Meals

As previously noted, carbohydrate digestion begins in the mouth with the secretion of the enzyme ptyalin. This enzyme, mixed with saliva, is crucial to proper digestion of carbohydrates. Food chewed into small particles is then completely mixed with a saliva/enzyme mixture to begin digestion. When food is swallowed after only a few short chews, as so many of us busy people do, there is insufficient time for ptyalin to do its job. Consequently, carbohydrate digestion is impaired. Large, inadequately chewed food

> In addition to chewing food thoroughly, care should be taken to restrict fluid intake with meals, as over-consumption of liquids may dilute digestive enzymes and HCl, thus impairing digestion.

particles are harder for the body to digest and can result in gas, bloating and indigestion.

Improper Food-Combining

Of the many food-combining rules that have been proposed, two emerge as most important in terms of their impact on the greatest number of people. These two rules are: (1) *Eat fruits alone or leave them alone* (Fruit is most beneficial when eaten 20 to 30 minutes before other food.) and (2) *Do not combine proteins and starchy carbohydrates at the same meal*. Disregarding these rules can slow down digestion, resulting in much gas and bloating. Here's why: Fruit is digested very rapidly when eaten alone because it is not digested in the stomach but rather is pre-digested, being high in enzymes. Fruit (especially melons) passes through the stomach in a very short period of time, 20 to 30 minutes, releasing nutrients in the intestine. If eaten with (or after) other foods, then fruit will not be able to move through the digestive tract as rapidly as usual since other foods, especially proteins, have a much longer transit time. (Meat, for example, has a transit time of as much as 6 hours.) Fruit will ferment if eaten last since other foods will block its passage through the digestive tract. The result could be gastric distress.

Combining proteins (like meat) with heavy starches (like pasta or potatoes) may not pose a problem for a person with a strong digestive system; however, this combination places a heavy demand on the output of both proteolytic (protein-digesting) enzymes and amalyse (starch-digesting), stressing the digestive system. Those with weak digestive systems may want to avoid these combinations. While separating proteins and starchy carbohydrates is desirable for those who have a slow **metabolism** (slow transit time), those who are **hyper-metabolic** (have a fast transit time) – about 20% of the population – will

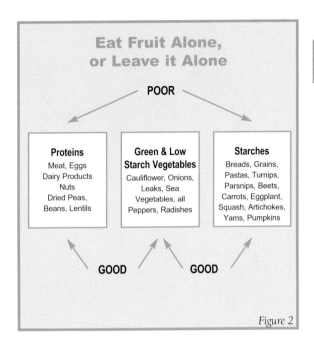

Figure 2

actually benefit from this combination because it will help to slow their metabolic rate.

These food-combining rules are most important to immune-compromised people with delicate digestive systems. Others, with good health, a hardy constitution and strong digestive organs may be able to disregard these rules without experiencing ill effects. It may be wiser therefore to view them as 'guidelines' rather than 'rules.'

Over-Eating

Overindulging in even the most nutritious foods will reduce their benefits, for the body will be unable to use the nutrients. Today, there is a virtual epidemic of obesity due in large part, undoubtedly, to the nutrient deficiency of the Standard American Diet (SAD). Nutrient imbalances and deficiencies may cause people to select foods unwisely. Overeating may be largely the mind's unconscious effort to satisfy the body's hunger for the missing nutrients (lost during processing and preparation).

The habit of frequent snacking results in an energy drain on the digestive organs, which can decrease their effectiveness and even have the net effect of shortening lifespan. This is substantiated by two rat studies done independently in the U.S. and Germany in the early 1970s. "Both groups found the rats fed but once a day had a lower body weight and higher enzyme activities in the pancreas and fat cells. It was also found that the life-span of the controlled eaters was longer by 17%."[2]

CLINICAL IMPLICATIONS OF IMPAIRED DIGESTION

Low Production of Hydrochloric Acid

Hydrochloric Acid (HCl) is a digestive acid produced in the stomach by millions of parietal cells that line the stomach. HCl is so strong that it will burn your skin. The lining of the stomach is protected from this acid, however, by a layer of mucus. Adequate production of HCl is critical to good health and a properly functioning digestive system because it:

- Helps break down protein
- Sterilizes food by destroying bacteria and microbes that are present
- Is required for production of **intrinsic factor** (needed for B12 absorption)
- Is needed for mineral absorption
- Signals the pancreas to secrete enzymes in the small intestine

HCl is critical in the digestion of protein. It breaks apart the chains of amino acids (protein constituents, which look like strings of pearls). Its presence also signals the production of pepsin, a protein-splitting enzyme, which further ensures that the amino acids are split into shorter chains to complete the process.

> **Some studies have found that 50% of the people older than 60 have low stomach acid.**

Indigestion, heartburn and ulcers are often thought to be caused by an over-production of stomach acid (hydrochloric acid). This is a common misconception. There is very little correlation between stomach acid production and these common digestive symptoms. In other words, you may experience heartburn or indigestion if you produce too much or not enough stomach acid. What is troubling is that physicians often treat chronic indigestion and heartburn with drugs that lower production of stomach acid. Some of these common drugs are Prilosec®, Zantac®, Tagament®, Pepcid®, Prevasid® and Nexium. In fact, the largest selling drug in America (and the world) is Prilosec. While decreasing production of stomach acid may relieve the symptoms of indigestion and heartburn, this may worsen the condition in the long term. This is particularly true if the underlying cause of indigestion and heartburn is an under production of stomach acid. There are many studies that have found that as we age hydrochloric acid production decreases by as much as 50%. When we do not produce enough stomach acid to digest our foods, or we eat too

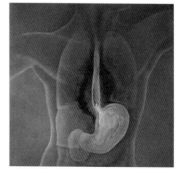

much food at one sitting, heartburn and indigestion are often the result. Prior to the 1960's, it was common for physicians to prescribe betaine hydrochloride for

2

Test Your pH

One way to determine if you have a HCl deficiency is to use special pH testing paper (which measures acidity/alkalinity) first thing in the morning to obtain a reading of the pH of your saliva. Record the number corresponding to the color change on the paper, then test the saliva again about 1/2 hour after eating breakfast. You should see an increase in pH, ideally by two whole numbers (from a pH of 7 to a pH of 9, for example). If the second reading decreases instead of increasing, and/or if the first reading was initially low (less than 6.5), it is an indication of a need for more stomach acid.[5]

Figure 3

cases of indigestion or heartburn. I have personally found this to be effective at relieving heartburn and indigestion. Until the mid-1990's, many physicians still believed that ulcers were caused by an over-production of stomach acid. It is now commonly known that the bacteria H. pylori is a common cause of stomach ulcers, and physicians now use antibiotics to treat ulcers. The message is clear. Hydrochloric acid is needed for adequate digestion of foods.

We constantly eat food that contains these microbes. There is no way to know if food prepared and served at restaurants is properly washed or if the water is clean. So, when the HCl level is low, there is a greater possibility of parasitic infestation. Another problem that can occur when HCl levels are low is vitamin B12 deficiency. HCl aids in the production of **intrinsic factor** in the stomach. Intrinsic factor binds with extrinsic (from food)

B12 to enable the absorption of B12 in the intestines. The lowering of stomach acid with age can inhibit the production of intrinsic factor and thus the absorption of B12. Many senior citizens have B12 deficiencies, which can result in muscle weakness and fatigue.

Other problems with low HCl include poor mineral absorption and reduced enzyme production. The presence of HCl in the duodenum signals the pancreas to release water, bicarbonate and enzymes. When the pH of the stomach is elevated or alkaline (due to HCl deficiency), the pH of the rest of the body can become imbalanced. The body cannot maintain homeostasis under these conditions, and serious degenerative diseases, including cancer, congestive heart failure, osteoporosis and Alzheimer's disease, can result.[3]

The symptoms of HCl deficiency are basically the same as those of excessive HCl production. These symptoms include:

- Bad breath
- A loss of taste for meat
- Stomach pain
- Fullness, distension in the abdomen
- Nausea/vomiting
- Gas
- Diarrhea and constipation
- Severe heartburn
- Intestinal parasites or abnormal flora
- Iron deficiency
- Itching around the rectum
- Undigested food in the stool
- Acne
- Candida infections
- Food allergies
- Weak, peeling and cracked fingernails[4]

Antacids…The Solution or the Problem?

When these symptoms are treated with antacids, there may be initial relief, but more problems eventually result. Antacids inhibit the body's

natural ability to pro-
duce HCl. As noted,
HCl has many benefits,
including sterilization of
our food. Without
enough HCl, uncon-
trolled growth of every
kind of microorganism
in the stomach such as
yeast, fungi and bacte-
ria can result. Antacids
alkalize the lower stom-

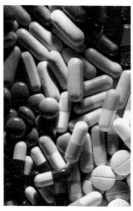

ach, triggering the release of more acid, requiring
more antacids. A vicious cycle occurs, with the
stomach alternating from too much acid production to not enough. This will eventually exhaust
the cells of the stomach, and they will become
unable to produce stomach acid.

Many antacids contain aluminum compounds,
which can bind the bowels, accumulate in
the brain and could be a factor in the eventual
development of Alzheimer's disease. Aluminum-
containing antacids can also cause long-term
depletion of the calcium stored in the body,
contributing to osteoporosis. Taking a medication
for heartburn that could cause ulcers, create an
overgrowth of yeast and bacteria, contribute to
Alzheimer's disease and damage the bones in the
body is not a good solution. A more natural
approach to the problem of low HCl would be to
take HCl supplements. More on that later.

Pancreatic Insufficiency

Besides secreting water and bicarbonates into the
duodenum to neutralize the acidity of chyme, the
pancreas also secretes **enzymes**, which break
down carbohydrates, protein and fats. Enzymes
that convert proteins (into amino acids) are the
proteases. Part of the job of protease enzymes is
to prevent allergic reactions resulting from the
absorption of non-digested protein, which causes an immune response in the lymphatic tissue of

the intestinal tract. Fifty percent of the body's
lymphatic tissue lines the intestinal tract to protect us from microbial invaders and toxins.

Poor production of pancreatic juice is termed
pancreatic insufficiency. The condition can
result from aging, physical and mental stress,
nutritional deficiencies, a diet of only cooked
foods, exposure to toxins or radiation, genetic
weakness, drugs and infection. Low HCl production will also inhibit pancreatic secretions.

Pancreatic insufficiency is an underlying cause of
high blood sugar (**hyperglycemia**). It is commonly found in people with **candidiasis** (an overgrowth of the yeast germ **Candida albicans**) and
those with parasite infections. Symptoms of
pancreatic insufficiency include gas, indigestion, abdominal discomfort, bloating, food sensitivities and the presence of undigested fat
(and other food) in the stool.[6]

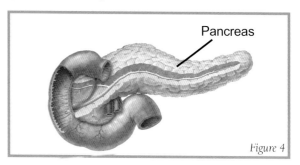

Pancreas

Figure 4

Lowered Enzyme Production

Enzymes are complex proteins that cause
chemical changes in other substances. They are the
basis of all metabolic activity in the body,
facilitating more than 150,000 biochemical
reactions and empowering every cell in the body to
function. There are three types of enzymes in the
body: **metabolic**, **digestive** and **food enzymes**.
Metabolic enzymes run and heal the body, giving
structure to **macronutrients** (fats, carbohydrates,
protein) and repairing damage. The body cannot
function or heal without metabolic enzymes.

The Role of Digestive Enzymes

The Enzyme

Protease	**Converts**	Proteins	**into**	Amino Acids
Lipase	**Converts**	Fat	**into**	Fatty Acids
Amylase	**Converts**	Carbohydrates	**into**	Sugars

Figure 5

Changing pH in the Body

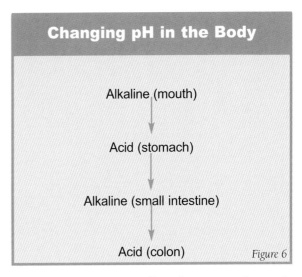

Figure 6

Digestive enzymes are manufactured by the pancreas. There are about 22 pancreatic enzymes, chief of which are **protease** (digests protein), **lipase** (for fat digestion) and **amylase** (for carbohydrate digestion). **Food enzymes** also digest food; however, they are supplied to the body solely through the diet, only from raw foods. These raw foods supply enzymes to digest the food in which they're found, with no extras to digest other foods.

Cooking at temperatures more than 116 degrees destroys food enzymes. Enzyme deficiencies are widespread in the American culture because virtually all food in the standard diet is refined (heat has been applied during processing).

Imbalanced Intestinal pH
pH is a measurement of acidity/alkalinity. It is measured on a scale from 0 to 14, with substances becoming increasingly more alkaline as the number increases, as per the following table:

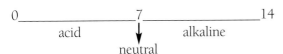

The optimal pH for digestion varies throughout the digestive tract as food moves through it. In the healthy digestive tract, the saliva secretes alkaline juices into the mouth; the stomach produces acid secretions; the pancreas and gallbladder discharge

alkaline juices to buffer the stomach acid; therefore, the small intestine is alkaline, and the colon is normally acid due to the presence of large populations of bacteria. So, there is a pH shift: alkaline (mouth) to acid (stomach) to alkaline (small intestine) to acid (colon).

An imbalance of intestinal **pH** can result from impairment of digestive secretions such as HCl and from pancreatic insufficiency. Lowered HCl production can result in an alkaline (rather than an acid) stomach. Pancreatic insufficiency could create an acidic (rather than an alkaline) environment in the small intestine if the pancreas fails to produce bicarbonate to alkalize the chyme leaving the stomach and entering the duodenum. Antacids can further complicate matters if taken habitually in an attempt to decrease heartburn.

If the pH of any of these key digestive organs is incorrect, the result will be incomplete digestion and its adverse health consequences.

Food Sensitivities
The improper digestion of food (especially proteins) can lead to an allergy-like response. When undigested food particles enter the lymphatic system through the walls of the intestine,

the body responds as if they were foreign invaders, known as **antigens**. An immune attack begins with the body producing **antibodies** (chemical bullets), which bind to the antigens, forming what are known as immune complexes. When this occurs, there may be enough of an immune system imbalance to create indigestion. In addition, stress can create a **sympathetic dominance** (fight or flight syndrome), which impairs digestion. Both of these responses can increase intestinal permeability and lead to more **food sensitivities**.

As the breakdown of the digestive and elimination processes occurs, an adverse reaction to any food can result. Certain foods show up more often than others as 'allergens.' These include milk, soy, wheat, corn, yeast, sugar, eggs and the 'nightshade' family, which consists of white potatoes, eggplant, tomatoes, chili peppers and garden peppers. Tobacco and certain drugs are also included in the nightshade category. Among the drugs so categorized are those containing atropine, belladonna and scopolamine, found in most sleeping pills.[7] It is important to know that a sensitivity or allergy to *any* food can develop, regardless of nutritional value or lack of it. It is also important to distinguish between an allergy and sensitivity.

Food allergies are easy to recognize. They involve immediate, strong reactions to foods, whereas a sensitivity expresses itself in a much more subtle way. Food sensitivities are delayed reactions to foods, which can occur anywhere from a few hours to a few days after exposure. With the allergic 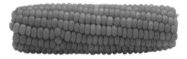 response, the areas of the body affected by exposure to the allergen are generally limited to the air passages, skin and digestive tract. When someone eats strawberries and develops hives, or is exposed to pollen and starts sneezing, this is a classic allergic

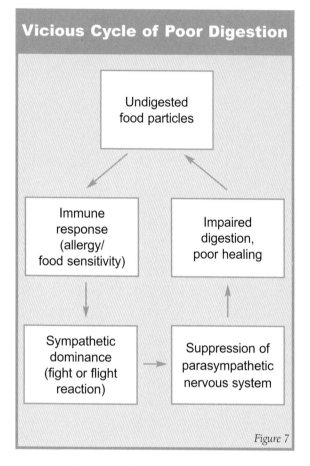

Vicious Cycle of Poor Digestion

Undigested food particles

Immune response (allergy/ food sensitivity)

Impaired digestion, poor healing

Sympathetic dominance (fight or flight reaction)

Suppression of parasympathetic nervous system

Figure 7

response, the type for which allergists test with skin prick tests. This type of reaction is an IGE antibody mediated reaction to antigens in the food. This is an acute **allergy**.

The IGG (as distinct from IGE) antibody reaction to food is generally known as a food sensitivity rather than a food allergy. The delayed food **sensitivity**, in contrast to the acute allergy, may affect *any* organ or tissue of the body, resulting in a wide array of physical and emotional symptoms. Such reactions, because they are delayed (by as much as three days), are frequently not recognized as food sensitivities. It is common for reactive foods to be consumed

Effects of the Sympathetic and Parasympathetic Systems on Selected Organs

Effector	Sympathetic System	Parasympathetic System
Pupils of eye	Dilation	Constriction
Sweat glands	Stimulation	None
Digestive glands	Inhibition	Stimulation
Heart	Increased rate and strength of beat	Decreased rate and strength of beat
Bronchi of lungs	Dilation	Constriction
Muscles of digestive system	Decreased contraction (peristalsis)	Increased contraction
Kidneys	Decreased activity	None
Urinary bladder	Relaxation	Contraction and emptying
Liver	Increased release of glucose	None
Penis	Ejaculation	Erection
Adrenal medulla	Stimulation	None
Blood vessels to:		
Skeletal muscles	Dilation	Constriction
Skin	Constriction	None
Respiratory system	Dilation	Constriction
Digestive Organs	Constriction	Dilation

Chart taken from *The Human Body in Health and Disease* by Memmler, Cohen, Wood, p. 148

Figure 8

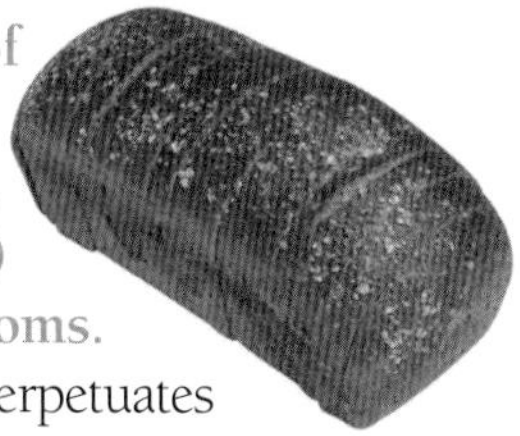

frequently, to the point of addiction, for by consuming such foods habitually, the body (unconsciously) avoids withdrawal symptoms. Unfortunately, this also perpetuates digestive disorders. When sensitive foods are eaten daily, the small intestine responds to the offenders by producing an antibody/antigen response. With the passing of time, this response irritates the digestive lining by producing inflammation. The response is analogous to wearing wool every day against the outer skin.

The skin would eventually react by becoming inflamed. The same holds true for the intestinal lining of the gut.

If people avoid the foods to which they're sensitive, they may start to feel somewhat better, but if digestion isn't improved, they will develop new sensitivities. On the other hand, if digestion is improved and toxins eliminated, sensitivities and allergies will be decreased or eliminated.

Both sensitivities and allergies can develop in response to anything in the environment – not just food. The response to the antigen – be it corn or petrochemicals – can affect any organ of the body. The gut will always be involved, however. Poor digestion is both the cause and the ultimate result of the allergic response or sensitivity, as figure 7 indicates. Significant stress will definitely lead to sympathetic dominance (see figure 8). This decreases digestive efficiency (less enzymes, etc.) and increases intestinal permeability, setting the stage for food allergies or sensitivities. The more food allergies or sensitivities, the more reactive the immune system becomes, creating more and more circulating antigen/antibody complexes. These will promote inflammation throughout the body, especially in the GI tract, creating further problems.

With food allergies and sensitivities, there is an element of increased permeability (leaky gut) of the intestinal tract that plays a dominant role in initiating the process. Undigested food particles have the effect of initiating an immune response, (allergic reaction) when they have made their way into the bloodstream. This can occur only when the lining of the intestine becomes porous. This condition of increased permeability or porosity of the lining of the intestine is known as 'leaky gut syndrome.'

Notes

[1] Michael Murray, ND, *The Healing Power of Foods*, Prima Publishing, 1993, p. 83.

[2] Dr. Edward Howell, *Enzyme Nutrition*, Avery Publishing Group, Inc., 1985, p. 112.

[3] Judy Kitchen, "Hypochlorhydria: A Review – Part 1," *Townsend Letter for Doctors and Patients*, October 2001, p. 56.

[4] Ibid., p. 58.

[5] Ibid.

[6] Elizabeth Lipski, MS, CCN, *Digestive Wellness*, Keats Publishing, Inc., 1996, p. 207.

[7] James Braly, MD, *Dr. Braly's Food Allergy and Nutrition Revolution*, Keats Publishing, Inc., p. 437.

Chapter Summary

Stress, broadly defined as anything that causes an extra load on the body, can be viewed as the cause of digestive dysfunction. Digestive stress comes in many forms, which may include:

- Emotional or physical stress
- Poor diet
- Medications
- Environmental toxins
- Over-consumption of processed food

If stress from any of these sources continues for an extended period of time, the result is a burdened digestive system and stressed supporting organs (such as liver and pancreas). The end result is altered function or structure of the body's organ systems which develops into:

- **Deficiency of HCl**, needed to break down proteins and protect from harmful microorganisms
- **Pancreatic insufficiency** (reduced enzyme and bicarbonate secretion), a precursor to more serious disease
- **Imbalanced intestinal pH**, which prevents proper digestion of foods due to excessive acidity or alkalinity of digestive juices
- **Food sensitivities and allergies**, which can be both the cause and the result of poor digestion

All of these stressors impair the digestive process, which leads to **intestinal toxemia** (the subject of the next chapter), Candida and parasites, an imbalance of gut flora, leaky gut and chronic disease, subjects of the next several chapters.

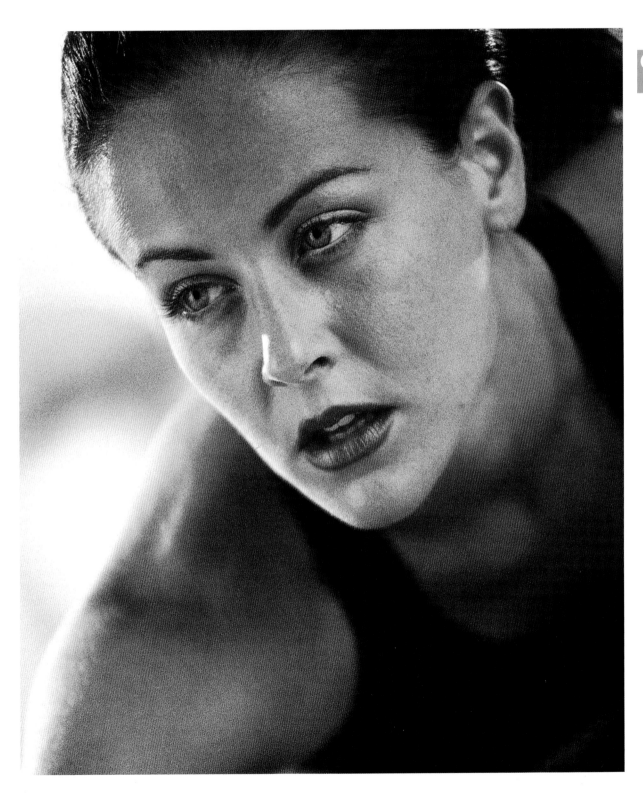

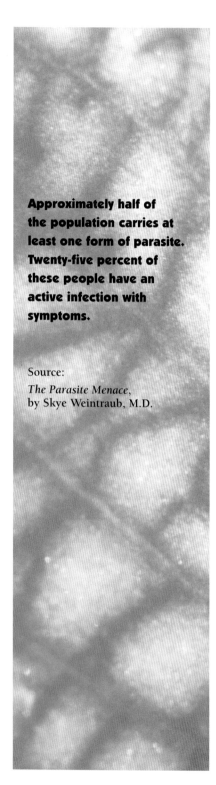

CHAPTER 3

EFFECTS OF digestive DYSFUNCTION

INTESTINAL TOXEMIA

Intestinal toxemia, poisoning of the intestines, occurs when the bacteria present in the gut act upon undigested food. This interaction can produce toxic chemicals and gases. These toxins, in turn, can damage the mucosal lining, resulting in increased intestinal permeability (leaky gut). The net result is that the toxins are then able to spread throughout the body via the bloodstream. In the words of Dr. John Matsen, ND, "If you don't digest your food quickly, some microorganisms will digest it for you, making toxins."[1] The waste products from these microorganisms produce some extremely potent toxins, 78 known types, including skatoles, indols, phenols, alcohol, ammonia, acetaldehyde and formaldehyde.[2] All of these are examples of **endotoxins**, internally produced toxins. They are just as damaging to the body as external environmental toxins, **exotoxins**.

Intestinal toxins can also produce **free radicals**, molecules with unpaired electrons, which cause damage to cells when they rip electrons out of cell membranes. Free radicals live only momentarily, but can do a great amount of damage in that short period of time. Large numbers of free radicals are produced by dozens of intestinal toxins. When the body is unable to buffer them due to toxic overload, disease results. To inactivate free radicals, the body deploys **antioxidants**, nutrients that act as free radical scavengers. Vitamins A, C and E and the minerals selenium and zinc are well known antioxidants. What is not so well known is that bile has even stronger free radical scavenging effects. This makes proper liver and gallbladder function important in preventing free radical damage.

In the beginning stages of intestinal toxemia, the body generally has sufficient nutritional reserves to manage the stress. At this point, it is not acutely distressed and may be without symptoms. However, as time passes, and the opportunistic organisms (bacteria, viruses, fungi, etc.)

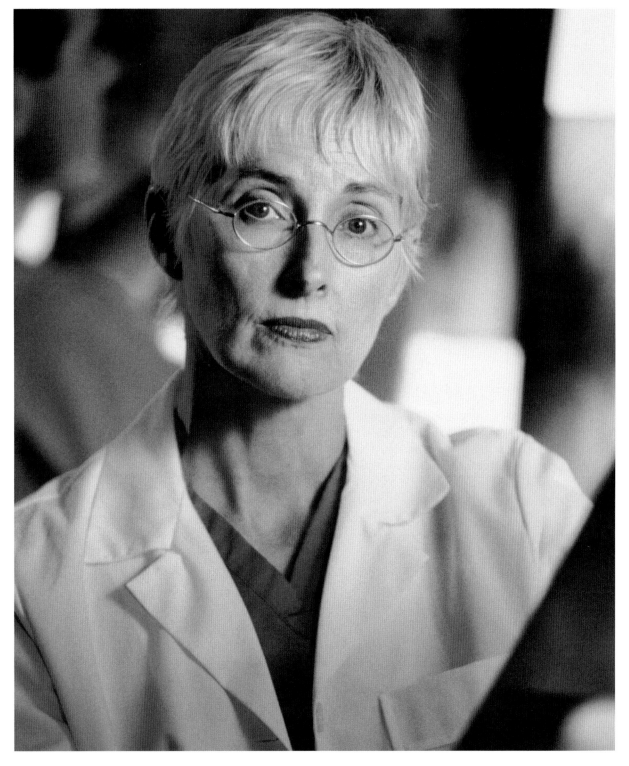

multiply, their toxic waste products overwhelm the body's defenses, transferring power from the 'good' to the 'bad guys.' As this happens, organisms that normally inhabit the GI tract in smaller numbers, without causing harm, such as parasites and Candida, can proliferate and produce symptoms such as gas, bloating, constipation, diarrhea, skin disorders, brain fog, chronic fatigue, irritable bowel syndrome and joint and muscle pain. These symptoms may or may not be recognized as the result of digestive stress, for they can occur anywhere in the body.

CANDIDA AND PARASITES – SECONDARY TOXIC SUPPRESSORS

Candida albicans, a yeast germ that becomes a problem when it proliferates and mutates to a fungal form, is actually a form of parasite, as are the other 'critters' that normally inhabit the GI tract – microorganisms like viruses, bacteria, worms, amoebas and protozoa. These are all considered 'secondary' toxic suppressors because of their opportunistic nature. They proliferate when the opportunity arises as a result of a shift in the body's terrain or internal environment (changes in pH, microbial population, muscular tone, etc.). Such a shift results in energetic and chemical imbalance, and may be caused by impaired digestion. The shift in terrain can also result from environmental pollution and drugs. Drugs and environmental toxins (non-steroidal anti-inflammatory drugs [NSAIDs], chemicals, solvents, metals, etc.), coupled with structural misalignments and emotional stress, may be viewed as primary toxic suppressors, in that they create an environment for the secondary toxic suppressors – the opportunistic microorganisms, which include Candida and parasites – to proliferate.

Candida and Other Fungi

Candida albicans is one of over 80 species of

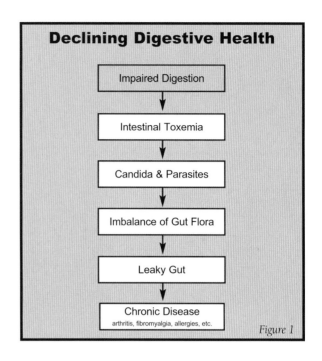

Declining Digestive Health

Impaired Digestion

↓

Intestinal Toxemia

↓

Candida & Parasites

↓

Imbalance of Gut Flora

↓

Leaky Gut

↓

Chronic Disease
arthritis, fibromyalgia, allergies, etc.

Figure 1

Candida and more than 250 species of yeast, many of which are parasitic in the human body. Candida is normally present in the intestinal tract in small amounts. When it remains in yeast form and exists in balance with the trillions of bacteria that normally inhabit the digestive tract, all is well with the body's internal eco systems. The ideal ratio of Candida to bacteria is 1:1 million; that is, 1 yeast to 1 million bacteria. This critical balance will be maintained if:

- The immune system is functioning normally.
- An optimal ratio of 'good'/neutral to 'bad' bacteria (80:20) is maintained.
- The pH of the colon is balanced (on the slightly acid side).

The medical community's awareness of Candida has been largely limited to the local effects of acute infection (candidiasis). Such infection involves invasion of the mucous membranes, typically on the skin, in the mouth ('**thrush**') and in the vagina ('yeast' infection). A chronic overgrowth of Candida in the intestines leads to an actual change in the form and function of the organism: It mutates from its yeast-like state to a fungal form. As such, Candida can lead to a variety of conditions that can affect the body physically and mentally – a fact not well recognized or accepted in traditional medical circles.

While many physicians still treat a vaginal yeast infection as a localized problem, a growing number are becoming aware that such infection is invariably accompanied by an overgrowth of Candida in the gut. To successfully resolve vaginal yeast problems and prevent their return, it is necessary to restore healthy conditions in the intestinal tract.

In its fungal state, Candida grows very long roots, **rhizoids**, which actually puncture the mucous lining of the intestine. It also secretes acid, which

Conditions That May Arise From Fungal Toxins

- Chronic fatigue
- Depression and anxiety
- Infertility
- Miscarriage
- Skin problems
- Arthritis
- Intestinal disorders
- Digestive problems
- Migraine headaches
- Sugar cravings
- Nutritional deficiencies due to malabsorption
- Hormone imbalances
- Jock itch
- Fingernail/toenail fungus
- Insomnia
- ADD
- Interstitial cystitis
- Respiratory disorders
- Fibromyalgia
- Heart conditions
- Multiple Sclerosis
- Female problems
- Allergies and environmental sensitivities
- Bladder infections
- Prostatitis
- Blurred vision
- Athlete's foot
- Ringworm
- Bad breath

Figure 2

can change the intestinal pH and can cause wear to this protective mucous lining. The resulting increased intestinal permeability is known as leaky gut syndrome. This condition permits the entrance of the fungus (and its toxic waste products) into the bloodstream along with other foreign substances and undigested food particles. This leads to a series of problems discussed in the 'Leaky Gut' section of this chapter.

Among the fungal toxins that can enter the bloodstream through the bowel wall is **acetaldehyde**, the major waste product produced by Candida. Acetaldehyde is a poison that is converted by the liver into alcohol. As alcohol increases (due to insufficient oxygen in body tissues), symptoms associated with drunkenness develop: disorientation, dizziness and mental confusion. The

Profile of a Killer Disease

Egypt, 1924: British egyptologist, Hugh Evelyn-White, was among the first to enter the tomb of King Tutankhamen, shortly after its discovery in 1922 near the ruins of Luxor. Evelyn-White became one of the dozen explorers to die soon after visiting the site. " I have succumbed to a curse," wrote he in his own blood in 1924, moments before hanging himself. At the time no one could explain his suicide nor the many other mysterious deaths of other unfortunate ones who had entered the tomb. Coming primarily to look for gold and treasures, the excavators paid no attention to the pink, gray and green patches of fungi on the chamber walls. So, in reality, King Tut's curse was a really severe allergic reaction to fungi: fruits and vegetables placed in the tomb to feed the pharaoh throughout eternity but which, decaying over centuries, had created deadly molds.

- from *Candida* by LucDe Schepper, MD, PhD, Lic. Ac., D.I. Hom, C. Hom.

poisonous effects of alcohol can result in anxiety, depression, irritability, headaches and fatigue. Acetaldehyde is just one of the Candida toxins involved in enzyme destruction, which results in impaired detoxification ability, decreased cellular energy production and a release of cell-damaging free radicals. There are thought to be more than 100 such toxins produced by Candida.

Candida toxins, carried to the liver by the bloodstream, proceed from there to other organs of the body – the brain, nervous system, joints, skin, etc. If the liver's detoxification ability is impaired due to inadequate nutrition and toxic overload, these toxins will be stored and can initiate chronic illness, including those conditions listed in figure 2.

Fungal toxins, known as **mycotoxins**, suppress immune function. Some of these toxins, like **aflatoxin**, have been linked to cancer and hardening of the arteries.

Of special interest to women is a mycotoxin called **zearalenone**, which mimics the effects of estrogen in the body. It is produced by a mold, **fusarium graminearum**, and is found primarily in corn products, bananas and in the meat of cattle fed contaminated corn. An overabundance of estrogen can result in such health problems as fibroids, breast lumps, infertility and cancer. The presence of zearalenone in the body can cause these problems as well. There are currently no limits placed on the amount of this mycotoxin permitted in grains intended for human consumption.[4]

Although the food supply is monitored for the presence of common mycotoxins, it is not uncommon for molds to contaminate grains and more commonly to affect nuts. Fungus is, in fact, ubiquitous in the environment – that is, found virtually everywhere. It is in the air and food. It even exists on exposed surfaces and can quite literally 'get under the skin.' Its presence in the skin appears to be aggravated by use of alkaline soaps.[5] Exposure to moldy environments can result in fungi and their toxins being introduced into the body. Fungal infections can also be transmitted sexually.

As previously mentioned, the presence of a small amount of yeast in the intestinal tract is normal, even helpful. However, it is abnormal for fungi to live inside the human body. Once inside, they live by ingesting dead or decaying matter.[6] Because fungal parasites must have sugar in order to survive, we often experience sugar cravings when harboring fungi. Giving in to those cravings only promotes more fungi.

Ironically, conditions that are caused by fungi are often medically treated with drugs (antibiotics, birth control pills, NSAIDs, cortisone) that destroy beneficial flora, thereby allowing fungi to proliferate, making the condition worse.

These drugs alter the terrain of the bowel by causing the extermination of good bacteria as well as bad. Any hormonal therapy, such as estrogen replacement, can cause an overgrowth of Candida in this manner. The elevation of progesterone during pregnancy and in the second half of every menstrual cycle may also stimulate Candida growth.

Candida secretes **carbon dioxide**, which may lead to gas and bloating. It is significant that poor

Drugs That Disrupt Intestinal Ecology

- Antibiotics
- Birth control pills
- Cortisone
- NSAIDs (non-steroidal anti-inflammatory drugs like ibuprofen)

Figure 3

digestion, which began the chain of events that led to Candida overgrowth, can also be an effect of it. Many people are caught in

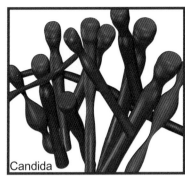
Candida

this vicious cycle. **It is very important that those with Candida overgrowth adhere to a special diet for a period of time. This diet is described in chapter 8. Those who experience some of the described symptoms should complete the adult or children's Candida self-analysis in the Appendix.**

Special laboratory tests for Candida are available through aware physicians. These tests include Candida antibody panels, intestinal permeability studies and digestive stool analysis. The International Health Foundation is a source for the names of physicians who are familiar with testing for and treating chronic systemic Candida infection. The Foundation's services are available at 901-660-7090 (http://candida-yeast.com). This non-profit organization, founded by pioneering Candida researcher/doctor, William G. Crook, MD, offers publications to direct people to health care professionals who are interested in yeast-related health problems.

> **It is said that 50% of the population is digesting and absorbing less than 50% of what we eat.**

Most nutritional practitioners know about Candida and the havoc it can create in the body. What isn't as well known is that Candida

Parasite News

Instead of experiencing better health, most of the people living in North America are deteriorating. People may be living longer, but they are not living healthier. There are many factors that contribute to this decline in health, but parasites may be one of the most overlooked.

The founding editor of *Prevention Magazine*, J.I. Rodale, once wrote an editorial stating that only those who protect themselves from the steadily increasing burden of toxic environmental pollution would survive in coming times.

infections often accompany parasite infections. The drain on the immune system by the parasite creates the opportunity for the Candida to proliferate. The following section explains the effect parasite infection can have on human health.

Parasites

Parasites have become a dominant health problem that many believe has reached epidemic proportions. It's something of a *silent* epidemic, however, because the problem is likely to go undiagnosed or be misdiagnosed. Some parasite problems have been recognized, even made headlines – like the outbreak of **Cryptosporidium** (a microscopic parasite) in the Milwaukee water supply in 1993, which made 400,000 people ill and killed 40. In that same year, parasite contamination was found in one out of every four municipal water supplies in 14 states. Cryptosporidium was featured on ABC News in the following year in reports that it had invaded New York City's water supply.

Another water-born parasite, **Giardia lamblia**, has been estimated by the Center for Disease Control to affect between 100,000 and 1 million people each year. In 1976, one of every six people in the U.S. was infected with one or more parasites.

In 1996, Dr. Omar Amin from Diagnostic Labs conducted a survey of 644 stool samples. In more than half (378), parasites were detected.[7] In the group, a number of typical characteristics emerged as shown in figure 4.

Parasite Survey Facts

- More than half the people with infection had traveled overseas in the past five years.
- People traveling to Mexico and Europe had the highest risk of infection.
- People living in households where someone was infected had twice the risk of infection.
- Of people infected, some had no symptoms.
- Some people unknowingly acted as carriers. (Since there are no symptoms, they could have been unaware, been untreated and passed parasites on to others.)
- People infected by more than one parasite had similar symptoms to those with single infections.
- Women were twice as likely to be infected as men and were more heavily infected.
- The most prevalent pathogens were E. histolytica, Giardia lamblia and Blastocystis hominis.[8]

Figure 4

Parasites are difficult to detect. They tend to hide in the lining of the intestines; and they live in other organs as well. If parasites are in the heart or lungs, they will not appear in the stool regardless of how well it's analyzed! Some of the reasons parasites are difficult to recognize and diagnose:

- Parasitic infestation has generally been considered a disease of the tropics, so a doctor isn't likely to consider it when making a diagnosis.
- Parasitology is seldom presented in mainstream medical journals or medical schools.
- Other than records of the Center for Disease Control, there is little tracking for parasites. With lack of information and little training, doctors aren't apt to look for parasites as an underlying cause of illness. If the symptoms aren't confined to the digestive tract, parasitic infestation could surely go undiagnosed.

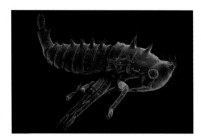

Parasites have a complex life cycle. Three of the most prevalent parasites found in the United States and worldwide shed at irregular intervals. This means that a parasite might be in the stool two to four days a week but not the rest of the week. If the person is tested for a parasite on a day it is not present, there will be a negative test result. The person would then go untreated. Therefore, it would be best for repeat stool samples (at least two to three) to be taken on non-consecutive days.

Another difficulty with parasite detection is there are many newly identified parasites that have not been sufficiently studied or recognized as pathogenic. An example would be **Cyclospora**, which was classified as a human parasite just a few years ago. The result of a parasite test done prior to the time that Cyclospora was recognized as pathogenic would have been reported as negative even though Cyclospora was present. By the 1990's, **Dientamoeba fragilis** was considered a pathogenic parasite though it had previously not been. The field of parasitology is thus evolving and continuously making discoveries of 'new bugs.'

Symptoms of Parasites

- Constipation/diarrhea
- Digestive complaints (gas, bloating, cramps)
- Irritability/nervousness
- Irritable bowel syndrome
- Persistent skin problems
- Granulomas (tumor-like masses that encase destroyed larva or parasite)
- Overall fatigue
- Disturbed sleep
- Anemia
- Muscle cramps
- Joint pain
- Post nasal drip
- Teeth grinding
- Prostatitis
- Sugar cravings & ravenous appetite
- Allergies

Figure 5

How do parasites threaten human health? They can injure the tissue of the digestive tract or most other organs. Most people don't realize this, but it is not only the parasite that can cause damage to the body, but also the waste that the parasite discharges into the body. This is part of the life cycle of any living organism: Food is ingested; waste is expelled. Parasites can disrupt the digestive process of the host, interfering with enzyme production and the breakdown of food. A properly functioning digestive system is critical to good health, so anything that disrupts this process will also affect the immune system. Remember: The mission of the parasite is to survive.

Degenerative disease can be associated with parasites. They create a mucous overlay in the gut that blocks absorption of nutrients so that the food we eat nourishes them, not us. Parasites can affect tissue anywhere in the body. Disorders that have been associated with parasites include arthritis, multiple sclerosis, appendicitis, both overweight and underweight conditions, cancer and epilepsy. Some cases of epilepsy have been associated with

pork tapeworm. This is probably due to auto-antibody production by the immune system in response to the parasites and the toxins they liberate. Pork should not be cooked in a microwave oven, as microwaves do not kill the **Trichinella** worm in it.

Parasites can get into the blood and travel to any organ, causing problems that are often not recognized as parasite-related. Consequently, disorders involving parasites are often wrongly diagnosed. A roundworm infestation in the stomach can give the appearance of a peptic ulcer. Amoebic colitis can be mistaken for ulcerative colitis. Tapeworms can be the unsuspected cause of blood sugar disorders, both **hypoglycemia** and diabetes. Their eggs, when present in the liver, can be mistaken for cancer. Those parasites that fall into the **protozoa** category can cause arthritis-like pain, as well as leukemia-like symptoms. Chronic Giardia

Parasite Sources

- Contaminated raw fruits and vegetables
- Raw or rare meat
- Polluted water/tap water
- Pets
- Vectors (carriers, like mosquitoes)
- Through the skin
- Through the nose (inhaled)
- Restaurant dining (especially at salad and sushi bars)
- Camping
- Previous parasite infection/reinfection
- Working in infant care
- Travel
- Solvents, like prophyl alcohol (alter internal terrain, making it suitable for parasites)
- Contact with someone who has parasites (a carrier)

Figure 6

can be an undetected element or missing diagnosis in both candidiasis and chronic fatigue syndrome.

The appendix has been described as the 'region of worms.' Due to its location at the bottom of the cecum, food residues and waste tend to accumulate and stagnate there, producing conditions favorable for parasites to thrive and appendicitis to develop.

Medical texts don't contain much information about parasites other than stating they can cause diarrhea and malabsorption. It is important to bear in mind, however, that parasites can mimic other disorders and/or produce no noticeable symptoms. When they do cause symptoms, a wide range can be displayed, as indicated in figure 5.

Another factor that no doubt contributes to the growing parasite epidemic is the widespread use of drugs that suppress immunity as a side effect. Many of the drugs in common use today are immunosuppressive and therefore increase our susceptibility to parasitic infection.

Although many external factors contribute to the parasite problem (see figure 6), by far the biggest factor is an internal one – a dirty colon, largely the result of an unwholesome lifestyle and bacterial imbalance in the colon.

IMBALANCE OF GUT FLORA

The flow chart in figure 1 shows how impaired digestion leads to intestinal toxemia (production

Causes of Intestinal Flora Imbalance

- Antibiotic use
- Refined carbohydrates
- Birth control pills
- Poor digestion/ elimination
- Stress
- Low fiber diet
- Steroid drug use
- X-rays/radiation therapy
- Chlorinated water
- Mercury toxicity
- Pollution

Figure 7

of toxins, as undigested food interacts with bacteria in the intestines). This toxemia, in turn, can lead to an overgrowth of harmful bacteria and often to Candida and parasites. Once these pathogens are established, they proliferate, and the bacterial imbalance is perpetuated, even increased, causing a vicious cycle.

The micro flora composition of the intestinal tract is complex. There are approximately 500 different species of micro flora that are part of the normal intestinal environment. There is a simple way to understand the different bacteria groupings in the gut: In every individual there is a ratio of **good** (health-promoting) bacteria, **neutral** bacteria (**commensal**) and **pathogenic** (disease-causing) bacteria. All of these organisms are competing for food and space in the digestive tract.

It is important that the good bacteria be abundant in the digestive tract. Bacteria become 'parasitic' if they do not remain in **symbiotic** relationship (harmony) with the rest of the microbial population. For example, if Candida (which is a natural inhabitant of the gut) or some other microbe grows out of control, the body is in a state of **dysbiosis**. Dysbiosis (out of symphony or 'disturbed biology') is a term coined by Dr. Eli Metchnikoff early in the twentieth century to describe an imbalance of intestinal flora and the accompanying conditions. Metchnikoff discovered the health benefits of probiotics and won the Nobel Prize in 1908 for his work with lactobacilli. He theorized that toxic compounds produced by bacterial breakdown of food were the cause of degenerative disease and a major factor in aging.

Beneficial flora are required for bacterial **fermentation** of dietary fiber, which results in **short-chain fatty acid** production. The short-chain fatty acids butyrate, acetate and lactate support the production of new cells, which is vital in rebuilding the intestinal tract. Where dysbiosis is present, the intestinal wall cannot be rebuilt, as it normally would be, every three to five days. An extra benefit of the short-chain fatty acids is the prevention of colon cancer.

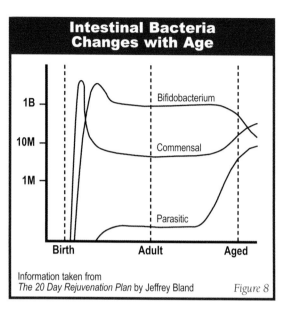

Intestinal Bacteria Changes with Age

1B

10M — Commensal

Bifidobacterium

1M

Parasitic

Birth   Adult   Aged

Information taken from
The 20 Day Rejuvenation Plan by Jeffrey Bland   *Figure 8*

known as 'small bowel dysbiosis,' a major cause of leaky gut syndrome. In addition, like the entire intestinal tract, the ICV muscular tone is controlled by the autonomic nervous system. When this system is imbalanced, a decrease in smooth muscle tone of the ICV could result in backflow of the colonic contents into the small intestine, again promoting leaky gut syndrome. Manipulation of autonomic nervous system balance may be helpful in providing normal intestinal tract tone and function. Modalities such as acupuncture, chiropractic manipulation, yoga and tai chi can be very helpful in this regard. The mechanics of the ICV and the recto-sigmoid portion of the colon can become compromised when the body is in the incorrect position for elimination of bowel contents. The correct posture would be a squatting position, which is the elimination posture used in much of the world.

Many factors cause dysbiosis, including poor diet, slow transit time and emotional stress. Chemicals and certain drugs can cause the condition, as can surgery and improper ileocecal valve (ICV) functioning. The ICV is the valve between the small intestine and large intestine. It is usually kept closed to prevent **reflux** (back flow) of fecal contents into the small intestine. Problems arise when constipation is present. As the peristaltic colonic waves attempt to propel the stool toward the rectum, backward pressure will push some of the liquid stool in the colon back through the ICV, causing contamination and colonization of the small intestine with colonic bacteria. This is medically

Where dysbiosis is present, the ideal ratio of beneficial to putrefactive (pathogenic) bacteria (80:20) is upset, even reversed. When **putrefactive** bacteria proliferate in the intestinal tract, peristalsis becomes sluggish. This inhibition of muscular contractions in the cecum causes food residues to concentrate in the appendix where they stagnate and cause inflammation (appendicitis = inflammation of the appendix).

There are many aspects of today's lifestyles that contribute to the destruction of beneficial flora, leading to dysbiosis (see figure 7). Dysbiosis commonly occurs due to faulty digestion, which results in partially digested food reaching the end

Good bacteria aids in:

- Digestion of food
- Absorption of nutrients
- Production of B vitamins
- Production of antibodies
- Destruction of competing bacteria

of the small intestine and entering the colon. The action of the colonic bacteria on partially digested food can result in the putrefaction of proteins and fermentation of carbohydrates, which may cause further growth of the pathogenic bacteria. This problem is greatly compounded when food stays in the intestinal tract too long (constipation).

LEAKY GUT

Toxic irritation of the gut lining is step two in our flow chart in figure 1. Intestinal toxemia is the direct result of impaired digestion caused by numerous stressors. This toxemia occurs when the bacteria that line the walls of the intestinal mucosa act upon undigested food. The toxins produced from this interaction attack the delicate intestinal mucosa, and allow for the development of systemic candidiasis and parasitic infection. Repeated attacks by these internally produced toxins (endotoxins) will, as time passes, erode the gut lining. This is the basic mechanism by which leaky gut develops. It can also be caused or aggravated by a number of other factors, as indicated in figures 10 and 11.

Factors Leading to Leaky Gut

- Alcohol (gut irritant)
- Caffeine (gut irritant)
- Parasites (introduced into the body by contaminated food and water)
- Bacteria (introduced into the body by contaminated food and water)
- Chemicals (in processed foods)
- Enzyme deficiencies (e.g. celiac disease, lactase deficiency, causing lactose intolerance)
- Diet of refined carbohydrates ('junk' food)
- Prescriptive hormones (like birth control pills)
- Mold and fungal mycotoxins (in stored grains, fruit and refined carbohydrates)

Figure 10

According to Elizabeth Lipski, MS, CCN, "NSAIDs (non-steroidal anti-inflammatory drugs) can cause irritation and inflammation of the intestinal tract, leading to **colitis** and relapse of ulcerative colitis … [They] can cause bleeding and ulceration of the large intestine and may contribute to complications of **diverticular disease** [outpouching of a segment of the intestine]."[11] Prolonged use of NSAIDs blocks the body's natural ability to repair the intestinal lining and also interferes with the production of prostaglandins, regulatory messengers that circulate throughout the body.

Drugs That Cause Leaky Gut

- NSAIDs (Non-steroidal anti-inflammatory drugs such as ibuprofen & aspirin)
- Antacids
- Steroids (includes prescription corticosteroids such as prednisone)
- Antibiotics

Figure 11

Unhealthy Digestive Tract

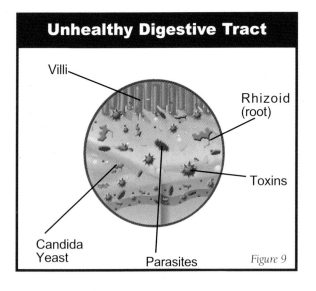

Villi

Rhizoid (root)

Toxins

Candida Yeast

Parasites

Figure 9

Autoimmune Diseases Resulting from Leaky Gut

- Lupus
- Rheumatoid arthritis
- Multiple sclerosis
- Chronic fatigue syndrome
- Fibromyalgia
- Crohn's disease
- Vasculitis
- Urticaria (hives)
- Raynaud's disease

- Alopecia areata
- Polymyalgia rheumatica
- Sjogren's syndrome
- Thyroiditis
- Vitilego
- Ulcerative colitis
- Diabetes

Figure 12

The mucous lining of the small intestine is a semi-permeable membrane that allows nutrients to enter the bloodstream, while shielding it from unwanted toxins and undigested food. This mucous lining is like the screen on a window in a house that lets the air in but keeps the bugs out. It is also like the skin, in that it sloughs off a layer of cells naturally every three to five days and produces new cells to keep the lining semi-permeable. Once endotoxins have eroded this membrane, however, it becomes permeable. (The 'screen' on the 'window' becomes filled with holes!) Now the toxins and food particles, which would normally not be permitted to enter the system, literally leak into the bloodstream. The body then becomes confused and attacks these unwanted toxins, as if they were foreign substances, and develops antibodies (chemical bullets) against them.

CHRONIC DISEASE

The net result of the above process is development of **autoimmune disease**, where the body makes antibodies against its own tissues. There are some 80 recognized autoimmune diseases (see figure 12 for a partial list); the cause of all of them is 'unknown' in medical circles.

Physicians are becoming increasingly aware of the importance of the GI tract in the development of autoimmune disease and allergy. In fact, "researchers now estimate that more than two-thirds of all immune activity occurs in the gut."[12] Allergies appear when the body develops antibodies to the (undigested) proteins derived from previously harmless food. These antibodies can enter any tissue and trigger an inflammatory reaction when that food is eaten. According to Zoltan P. Rona, MD:

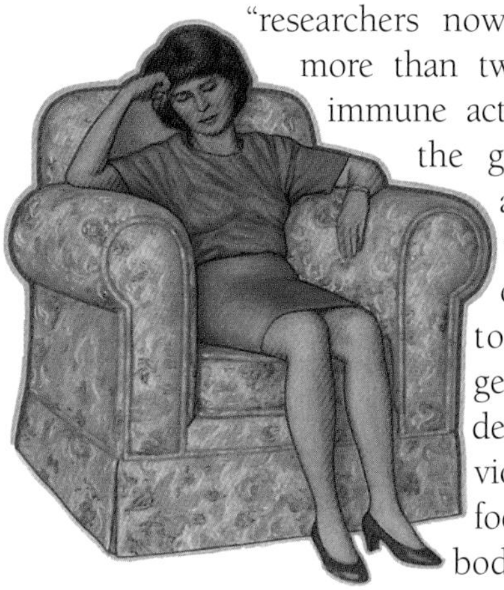

> If this inflammation occurs in a joint, autoimmune arthritis (rheumatoid arthritis) develops. If it occurs in the brain, myalgic encephalomyelitis (a.k.a. chronic fatigue syndrome) may be the result. If it occurs in the blood vessels, vasculitis (inflammation of the blood vessels) is the resulting autoimmune problem. If the antibodies end up attacking the lining of the gut itself, the result may be colitis or Crohn's disease. If it occurs in the lungs, asthma is triggered on a delayed basis every time the individual consumes the food which triggered the production of the antibodies in the first place.[13]

Leaky gut syndrome can cause malabsorption of many important nutrients – vitamins, minerals and amino acids – due to inflammation and the presence of many potent toxins. This malabsorption can also cause gas, bloating and cramps and eventually such complaints as fatigue, headaches, memory loss, poor concentration and irritability. The set of symptoms known collectively as **irritable bowel syndrome** (IBS) – bloating and gas after eating and alternating constipation and diarrhea – has also been linked to leaky gut syndrome, as has eczema.

Because of our high stress lifestyles, many of us have an overworked, under-functioning digestive system, imbalanced intestinal flora and a continuous flow of intestinal toxins seeping into the bloodstream. Why then do some people seem unaffected, able to eat or drink just about anything they choose, showing no ill effects, while others experience discomfort and ultimately chronic disease? The difference has much to do with the functioning of the gallbladder and the detoxification ability of the liver, presented in chapter 5. ✳

Notes

[1] John Matsen, ND, *The Mysterious Cause of Illness*, Fischer Publishing Corporation, 1987, p. 25.

[2] Ibid.

[4] Doug A. Kaufmann, *The Fungus Link*, Mediatrition, 2000, p. 155.

[5] Jack Tips, ND, Ph.D, *Conquering Candida*, Apple-A-Day Press, 1995, p. 37.

[6] Op. Cit., Kaufmann, p. 148.

[7] Trent W. Nichols, MD and Nancy Faass, MSW, MMPH, *Optimal Digestion*, Quill, 1999, p. 147.

[8] Ibid., p. 148.

[10] William Welles, DC, "The Importance of Squatting" (unpublished article).

[11] Elizabeth Lipski, MS, CCN, *Digestive Wellness*, Keats Publishing, Inc., 1996, p. 778.

[12] Wendy Marson, "Gut Reactions," *Newsweek*, November 17, 1997, p. 95–99.

[13] http://www.naturallink.com/homepages/zoltan_rona/leaky

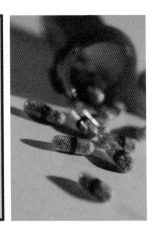

"...inflammation in the intestinal wall (called enteritis) ...develops in 70% of people taking NSAIDs daily for two weeks."

Leo Galland, MD, *The Four Pillars of Healing*

Chapter Summary

As our figure 1 flow chart indicates, impaired digestion leads to intestinal toxemia, wherein bacteria act upon undigested food in the gut, producing endotoxins. Intestinal toxemia can lead to an overgrowth of putrefactive bacteria and often Candida. Overgrowth of Candida is often accompanied by parasites. Proliferation of these opportunistic organisms further upsets the bacterial balance in the intestines. An overgrowth of pathogenic bacteria can cause irritation of the intestinal tract, tissue damage and impaired circulation, any of which can lead to gastrointestinal inflammation.

The intestinal wall cannot renew itself without sufficient beneficial flora to ferment dietary fiber into short-chain fatty acids. Leaky gut syndrome occurs when the mucosal lining of the intestinal tract becomes porous and irritated. As time passes, the breakdown in the intestinal mucosa can result in the passage of undigested food particles, toxins, parasites and Candida by-products into the bloodstream. This can lead to a weakened immune system, digestive disorders and, eventually, chronic disease.

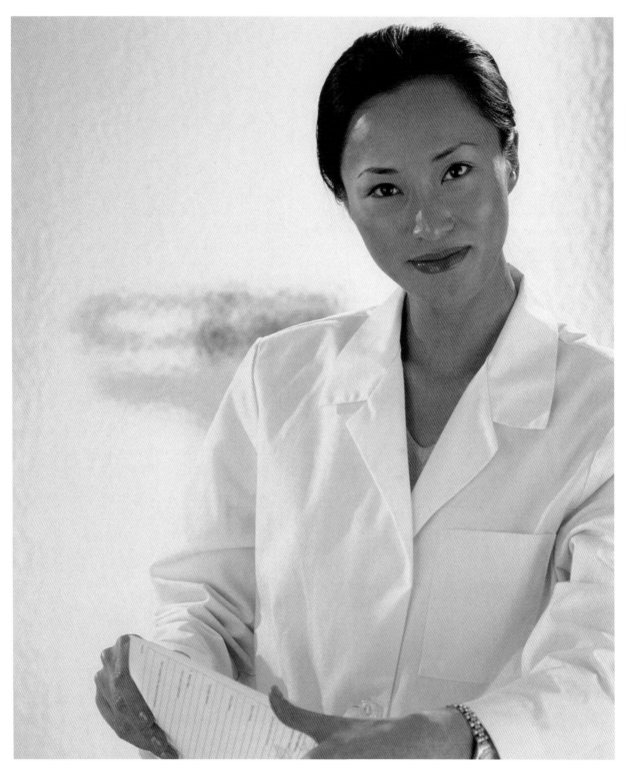

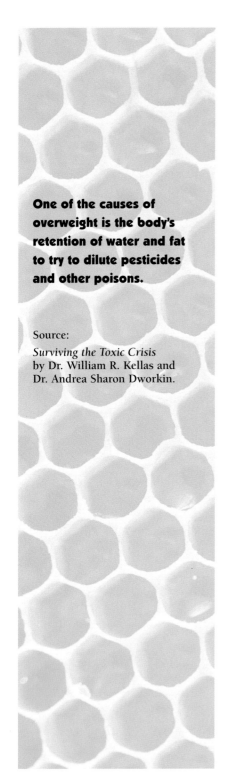

CHAPTER 4

TOXIC
suppressors

One of the causes of overweight is the body's retention of water and fat to try to dilute pesticides and other poisons.

Source:
Surviving the Toxic Crisis
by Dr. William R. Kellas and
Dr. Andrea Sharon Dworkin.

When the liver is overburdened with intestinal toxins, resulting from impaired digestion, its detoxification capacity (and that of other organs of elimination) is strained. The result is that toxins can be stored in fatty tissues of the body. When other sources of endotoxins are present, as well as major exotoxins (like drugs and chemicals), the detox capabilities of our livers are stressed to the maximum. The inevitable result is chronic disease.

This chapter presents information on the over-abundance of toxins in the environment and how the body manages this toxic load. Toxins are in our homes, workplaces, water and air. This is largely the result of technological advancement in the modern world. Agricultural chemicals are sprayed on and chemical additives are introduced into our food. More drugs are prescribed and taken than ever before. Today there are more than 1,000 drugs and chemicals that can injure the liver.[1] Perhaps more injurious than these individual drugs and chemicals is the effect of their interactions, which remains largely unknown.

We drink chlorinated and fluorinated water, and inhale pollutants like car exhaust, paint fumes and chemicals from clothes and carpets. No wonder the body has more toxicity than ever! The result of this toxic exposure is everything from chemical sensitivity to digestive problems to cancer! The following section describes some of the pollutants in our environment.

DRUGS

The term 'drugs' encompasses prescription and over-the-counter medications, as well as 'recreational' drugs. All drugs cause some side effects. Many drugs affect the organs of the digestive system, the accessory digestive organs and/or the organs of elimination, thus adversely impacting the digestive and/or eliminative functions of the body. As chemicals, drugs are basically toxins. While a controlled dose can have

4

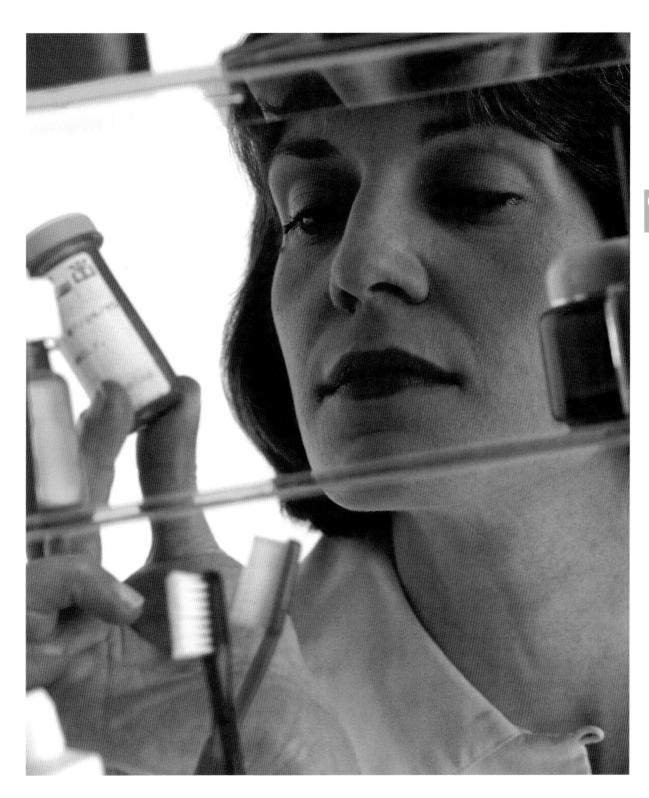

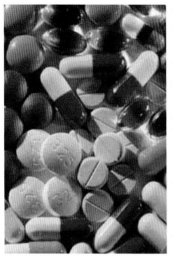

the effect of eliminating (often in the form of suppressing) symptoms, an overdose can have damaging, even fatal, effects. Many drugs can cause damage to the liver and/or kidneys, the body's primary and secondary eliminative organs, respectively. Physicians often monitor blood levels of powerful medicinal drugs to avoid such damage.

Constipation is another common side effect of many medications. It can result from ingestion of anti-depressants, pain medications, diuretics, antibiotics and antacids that contain aluminum. As previously noted, **antacids** can further aggravate the very symptoms they're taken to alleviate (heartburn, indigestion). They also inhibit phase I detoxification in the liver (discussed in chapter 5) and can cause damage to this organ. Constipation is but one of many symptoms that can result from **antibiotics**, which destroy both good and bad bacteria in the digestive tract. Antibiotic use can result in overgrowth of yeast and fungus with the attendant problems. Tetracycline use can cause development of fatty deposits in the liver. Erythromycin can cause **cholestasis** (diminished bile flow).

Listed below are other drugs (both medicinal and recreational) that can negatively affect the digestive/eliminative process:

Alcohol – Alcohol abuse can lead to cirrhosis of the liver, gastritis and pancreatitis. Alcohol use can destroy normal intestinal permeability.

Antihistamines – These drugs inhibit phase I detoxification in the liver.

Benzodiazepines (Halcion, Centrax, Librium, Valium®, etc.) – These drugs inhibit phase I detoxification in the liver.

Birth control pills – Their use can contribute to an increase in yeast due to an increase in unnatural progesterone; can increase risk of gallstones.

Caffeine – In some individuals and at some doses, caffeine can cause nausea, diarrhea and stomach pain. It also causes frequent urination, putting an extra load on the kidneys.

Cocaine – Its use can cause acute hepatitis.

Laxatives – Stimulant laxatives, even the herbal variety (such as senna and cascara sagrada), act by irritating the bowel, and they can be habit-forming. Many contain **psyllium**, a soluble fiber that absorbs 40 times its weight in water. This has the effect of dehydrating the bowel, which will aggravate the constipation problem rather than solve it. Pharmaceutical laxatives can also cause mineral depletion and lead to a 'leaky gut.' Laxative abuse can lead to kidney failure.

Marijuana – Although considered harmless by many, marijuana sets up conditions favorable to yeast growth. It lowers HCl production, which could allow the proliferation of the ulcer-causing bacteria H. pylori[2] and lead to a number of other systemic problems associated with HCl deficiency.

NSAIDs (non-steroidal anti-inflammatory drugs) – Classic NSAIDs, which include aspirin and ibuprofen, are prescribed to reduce pain and inflammation, but they directly irritate the lining of the stomach and can actually cause ulcers and lead to leaky gut syndrome. Aspirin can cause bleeding in the GI tract. If taken in large doses, or by sensitive individuals, aspirin may also damage the kidneys. These drugs inhibit the liver's phase II detoxification enzymes. The newer COX-II NSAIDs have less serious GI side effects but can still cause damage.

Steroids (cortisone, prednisone, anti-inflammatories) – Among the many side effects of these drugs is deterioration of the intestinal lining. Ironically, they are often prescribed for arthritis, an autoimmune condition *caused by* leaky gut. These drugs are also damaging to the liver.

Tobacco – There are 47 different toxins in cigarette smoke, including nicotine and toxic metals – nickel, cadmium, lead and arsenic. Nickel is actually the most allergenic and most carcinogenic metal to which we're exposed.[3] Among the symptoms of nickel allergy are autoimmune diseases such as lupus or arthritis, asthma, mucus

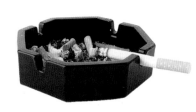

in the throat and nasal polyps. The gastrointestinal effects of cadmium poisoning include weight loss, vomiting, anorexia, diarrhea, constipation and abdominal pain. Exposure to high levels of cadmium can damage kidneys and liver. The metal has also been linked to emphysema.[4] Lead poisoning can cause the following gastrointestinal symptoms: nausea and vomiting, diarrhea or constipation, colic, abdominal rigidity and pain, loss of appetite and weight. Arsenic poisoning can result in similar gastrointestinal effects: anorexia, diarrhea, constipation, abdominal pain. It can also cause liver and kidney damage, hair loss, edema, dermatitis and blotchy, hardened skin.

Another component of cigarette smoke is carbon monoxide, which, at high levels, can cause asphyxiation. In smokers, it reduces the amount of oxygen available to the body. Cigarettes also contain tar, a carcinogen (cancer-causing substance) that clogs the alveoli in the lungs. There is also a higher incidence of liver cancer (and, of course, lung cancer) in smokers than in non-smokers.

People with liver diseases like hepatitis, alcoholic liver disease and **hemochromatosis** (a hereditary disease of iron overload) are hampered in their detox ability and must be especially careful with use of liver-damaging drugs and other chemicals. In high doses, the fat-soluble vitamin A (in its synthetic form) can pose a danger to the liver, especially in those with prior liver problems. Even herbs like valerian root, chaparral, kava kava and comfrey can cause damage in such sensitive people.

Chemotherapy and Radiation

Diagnostic radiation includes x-rays, along with the use of radioactive substances, like iodine and thallium, which are injected into the body. X-rays are a form of **ionizing radiation** – radiation that is powerful enough to knock electrons out of atoms. It can damage dividing cells, and in so doing, damage DNA. Ionizing radiation can also give rise to mutations inside cells, which ultimately leads to cancer – a condition that is, ironically, *treated* with irradiation. Radiation, in the form of x-rays, radioactive cobalt or radium, is used to destroy cancerous cells. The problem is that it also damages normal cells in the process.

Cancer is also treated with **chemotherapy**, a process that employs the use of cytotoxic drugs. These drugs, as their name implies, poison cells. Once again, while the intent is to target cancer cells only, there is frequently destruction of normal cells as well. The side effects of chemotherapy can be quite severe and varied as a result of damage to

4

organs and bone marrow. Although chemotherapy is an accepted and widely used form of treatment for cancer, "its effectiveness for many cancers is weak and in some cases nonexistent."[5] It is often used in conjunction with radiation. These two together constitute the 'standard of care' in cancer treatment in medical circles today, despite their unimpressive track record and the vast amount of suffering they have caused.

ORAL FOCAL INFECTION

Routine dental procedures that are invasive by nature, such as root canal therapy and tooth extractions, stress the entire body and can set the stage for microbial proliferation (and resultant toxic damage), giving rise to 'focal infection' in the oral cavity. A focal infection is chronic in nature and often hidden, as the symptoms it produces may be distant from the actual focal site. It is a walled off area of concentrated toxins where dead tissue or infection can be found.

When the nerve of a dying tooth is extracted and filling material is placed in the canal of the root (endodontic therapy), the bacteria present in that tooth and surrounding tissues take refuge in structures known as **dentin tubules**. There are literally miles of these tubules associated with every tooth site, and it is impossible to sterilize them. Bacteria from these sites, as well as their toxins, can travel to other areas of the body, creating problems. Details about the problems associated with root canal treatment can be found in Dr. George Meinig's classic book, *Root Canal Cover Up*.

A condition that most often accompanies a root canal filled tooth, and often occurs at an extraction site, as well, is known as a **jawbone cavitation**. A 'cavitation' (technically known as osteonecrosis – dead bone) is a hollow space in the jawbone. In the case of an extraction site, the area heals over superficially with gum tissue, but below the gum

surface is a hole or porous area in the bone. The formation of the cavitation is often the result of the dentist's failure to remove thoroughly the ligament 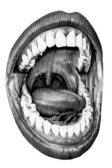 connecting bone to tooth when extracting a tooth. Bacteria from the ligament are trapped in the hollow space and mutate into virulent **anaerobic** forms (not requiring oxygen) since blood supply (and hence oxygen) to the site is severely limited. Like the root canal site, a cavitation is a focal point of infection that can spread toxicity via the bloodstream and lymphatic system to distant areas of the body. The toxins produced at cavitation sites are some of the most potent known. The condition is widespread, but underdiagnosed, since patients often have no symptoms in their mouths and do not realize that their systemic problems may be coming from a silent jawbone condition. Jawbone cavitations interfere with the production of enzymes critical to generation of energy in the body and thus can cause serious systemic problems. For more information on cavitations, read Susan Stockton's *Beyond Amalgam: The Hidden Health Hazard Posed by Jawbone Cavitations* (Power of One Publishing, 1-800-830-4778, ext. 246).

> "If your systemic problems have their origin in your mouth, no amount of symptomatic treatment will solve the problem. You can fast until the cows come home and follow all kinds of detoxification and nutrition programs. However, until you shut off the toxic fountain in your jawbone, you are not likely to take a significant step toward wellness."
>
> Susan Stockton, *Beyond Amalgam*

Where jawbone cavitations or other oral foci are present, *systemic detoxification efforts may be of limited success until the focus is removed* because the focal conditions often give rise to proliferation of opportunistic organisms such as Candida. Since fungi live on dead (necrotic) matter, cavitations provide them with an abundance of food, a feast of dead bone. Until this food source is removed by elimination of the focus (surgical removal of the dead bone), the fungi cannot be successfully eliminated.

Jawbone cavitations and root canal sites may be considered primary toxic stressors as may toxic metals, such as nickel and mercury, that are placed directly into the tooth structure. Metal crowns, bridges and mercury-containing amalgam ('silver') fillings are examples. The presence of heavy metals in the teeth (and consequently in the jawbone) will make it difficult to rid the body of secondary toxic suppressors like Candida and parasites: The first order of business is to eliminate the heavy metals and oral foci; then the way will be clear to address the parasite problem.

Many biological dentists are trained to recognize and treat focal infections. DAMS (Dental Amalgam Mercury Syndrome), which can be contacted at 1-800-311-6265, is a source for names of such dentists, as well as those who have mercury-free practices.

ENVIRONMENTAL TOXINS

Doctors Kellas and Dworkin, in their book, *Surviving the Toxic Crisis*, originally made the distinction between **primary toxic suppressors** and **secondary toxic suppressors**.[6] Among the primary toxic suppressors already noted are drugs, focal infection and emotional stress. Structural misalignment is another primary toxic suppressor, for when certain vertebrae in the spine are misaligned, they interfere with nerve supply to

Primary Environmental Toxins

- Electromagnetic pollution
- Chemicals/solvents
- Metals
- Air/water pollution

Figure 1

4

digestive organs, causing dysfunction. Environmental toxins are also primary toxic suppressors. These consist broadly of electromagnetic pollution, chemicals/solvents, metals and air/water pollution.

These influences allow secondary toxic suppressors to flourish after the primary damage has been done. The secondary toxic suppressors are parasites. These include yeast and fungi, amoebas, protozoa, bacteria, viruses and worms.

Electromagnetic Pollution

Electromagnetic pollution is a very broad term that encompasses those frequencies emitted from electrical and electronic devices, which can have a damaging effect upon the body. These include ionizing forms of radiation, such as x-rays, gamma rays and ultraviolet radiation. The ill effects of these frequencies are well known. Not so well known are the problems that can arise from exposure to radiations lower on the electromagnetic spectrum, such as microwaves and **extremely low frequencies (ELFs)**.

Russian, German and Swiss researchers have found many problems arising from the continual ingestion of microwave-cooked foods. These problems may result from the inability of the body to metabolize the unknown by-products produced by exposing foods to microwaves. Such exposure also reduces and/or alters the nutrients in food.[7] Among the adverse gastrointestinal effects of microwaves, as noted by the Russians, are stomach

pain and an increased incidence of appendicitis.[8]
Stomach and intestinal tumors, as well as immune
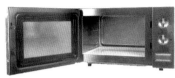 system deficien-
cies resulting from
blood and lymph
alterations, may
be among the
long-term effects.[9] Cell phones, in widespread use
today, also emit microwave radiation, much of
which is absorbed into the brain, posing a significant health risk.

ELFs are those frequencies less than 300 hertz or
cycles per second. They encompass the 60-cycle
current on which the standard electrical grid
system in the U.S. is based. The pioneering work
of Robert O. Becker, MD in the 1970s, demonstrated
the potentially adverse effects of being in continuous
proximity to a source of these frequencies. He
found that such exposure elicited a constant stress
response in animals, which led ultimately to lowered
immunity and all manner of disease.

Chemicals/Solvents

We have considerable exposure to fat-soluble,
carbon-containing, toxic chemicals used as solvents, glues and paints. Cleaning products,
formaldehyde, toluene and benzene are all 'solvents.' These fat-soluble chemicals collect in the
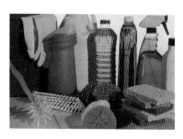 fatty tissues of the
body rather than
being excreted
quickly. They are
particularly dam-
aging to those
who are deficient
in essential fatty
acids, as "the oil-starved body will latch onto oily
substances (such as diesel exhaust) in much the
same way a dry sponge soaks up water."[10] These
compounds can cause liver and kidney damage as
well as skin irritation.

Cologne and personal care products (which can
cause asthma and skin rashes)[11], food additives,
(which can cause diarrhea, constipation, nausea,
lung changes, rashes)[12] and pesticides are also
'chemicals.' Pesticides cause a wide range of disorders affecting the organs of elimination and
digestion – constipation/diarrhea, liver and
kidney damage, bladder irritation, rashes and
wheezing[13] – though primary damage is to the
nervous system.

Metals

The earlier section about drugs (tobacco), noted
the damaging effects of nickel, lead, cadmium and
arsenic. These metals are very prevalent in the
environment, as indicated below:

Nickel is a component of stainless steel and therefore is found in such items as cookware and
inexpensive earring wires or posts and other jewelry made of stainless steel. Nickel is also found in
cosmetics, hydrogenated oils and fats, and
processed, refined foods. It is used in dentistry in
numerous restorative materials, including the
majority of porcelain crowns.

Lead can be found in tap water, pesticides, soft
coal, cigarette smoke, lead crys-
tal dishes and glassware, batteries, pewter ware, ceramic glazes,
liver, and some domestic and
imported wines. Other sources
include lead solder on cans,
as well as lead present in some hair dyes and
rinses, bone meal, insecticides, vinyl mini-blinds,
porcelain glazed sinks and tubs and pipes in
old buildings.

Cadmium is found in cigarette
smoke, tap water, galvanized
pipes, plastics, nickel-cadmium
batteries, fertilizers, fungicides,
contaminated air and soil, shellfish

found near industrial shores, coal burning and plastics. It is also present in most pink dyes used in dentistry to color dentures.

Arsenic is found in smog, laundry aids, insecticides, herbicides, rat poison, the manufacture of mirrors, some paints and dyes, contaminated seafood and kelp, wine, refined table salt and beer. It may also be found in store-bought grains due to rodenticide residue.

Two other toxic metals that are extremely prevalent in the environment today are aluminum and mercury. Aluminum toxicity can cause gastrointestinal irritation and can also lead to decreased liver and kidney function.

Almost all food and water supplies contain some amount of aluminum, for it is used by municipal water supplies as a 'flocculating' agent to remove dirt, and it is widely used in food processing. It is also found in cookware, foil and utensils, anti-perspirants, paints, cosmetics and baking powders, as well as in over-the-counter pain killers, anti-inflammatory drugs, antacids and douche preparations.

Mercury toxicity is of special interest, given the widespread use of the metal in dentistry. The 'silver' fillings commonly used are actually 50% mercury. The other 50% consists of other metals. Mercury vapors escape from these fillings every time food is chewed, poisoning the body.

Mercury is found in fish from contaminated salt water, in cosmetics, fluorescent lights, thermometers, barometers, fungicides, pesticides and some hair dyes. Some seeds are also treated with methyl mercury chlorine bleaches.

> "...amalgam leaches mercury continuously throughout the lifetime of the dental filling. Mercury vapor is the main way that mercury comes out of amalgam, and this vapor is absorbed at a rate of 80 percent through the lungs into the arterial blood. Mercury is more effective as a killer of cells (cytotoxity) than many cancer chemotherapies. There is no harmless level of mercury vapor exposure."
>
> **Morton Walker, DPM, *Elements of Danger***

Symptoms of mercury toxicity include loss of taste and smell, a metallic taste in the mouth, asthma, rashes, constipation, ulcers, bloating, gas and frequent night urination. Mercury toxicity can cause a string of negative effects in the digestive system, for it "combines with bile and can cause bile from the gallbladder to become more alkaline, providing a favorable environment for parasites. These parasites can plug up the hepatic or bile duct so that needed digestive and other enzymes from the gallbladder, liver and pancreas are not released. Gallbladder function then suffers."[14] With a blocked gallbladder, oils are not absorbed; therefore hormone production is lowered, and lymph cleansing is impaired. Also, oil deficiency encourages the body to absorb toxic petrochemicals.[15] Mercury is neurotoxic and cumulative in the system. It can interfere with the entry of nutrients into the cells and removal of wastes from them. It can also interfere with the normal immune response by binding with immune cells and destroying them.

All toxic metals have many ill effects. This presentation has been limited largely to adverse effects upon digestion and organs of elimination.

Heavy metal overload in the body can often be detected through hair analysis, a test performed by special labs. Natural health care providers have the details.

Air/Water Pollution

Pollution of air and water is a planet-wide phenomenon of staggering proportions. The World Health Organization reports that 90% of chronic illness is related to environmental factors.[16] Pollution affects the indoor as well as outdoor environment. In fact, the average indoor environment is actually *more* polluted, as it contains hazardous chemicals in concentrations 10 to 40 times greater than those outside.[17] Indoor pollution typically comes from formaldehyde, aerosol spray products, air fresheners, asbestos, microbes and mold spores, car-

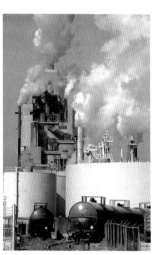

bon dioxide, house dust, cooking gas, colognes and cleaning products. In a poorly ventilated building, these pollutants are concentrated and can give rise to a number of symptoms. Major among the gastro-intestinal symptoms produced by such exposure is nausea. Chronic exposure to a highly contaminated indoor environment can result in chemically induced immune disorders (multiple chemical sensitivities and environmental illness). MCS and EI are common today due to widespread pollution, though often misdiagnosed. Dr. Gloria Gilbère, Director of the Naturopathic Health and Research Center in Bonners Ferry, ID, is a recognized authority on these subjects, as well as fibromyalgia and leaky gut. Her web site is www.drgloriagilbere.com. She can be reached at 208-267-5417.

Poor air quality in commercial airlines is receiving an increasing amount of attention these days. Due to poor ventilation, microorganisms and

Contaminants in Airplanes

- Carbon dioxide from breathing and dry ice
- Ozone from the earth's atmosphere
- Nitrogen oxides from jet fuel combustion
- Volatile organic compounds (VOCs) from fuel and cleaning fluids
- Fibers and dust
- Bacteria, fungi and viruses from food and passengers
- Tobacco smoke on international flights[18]

Figure 2

pollutants can build to dangerous levels. The ventilation systems used by airlines draw outdoor air through the engines. This air is mixed with recycled air from the cabin. More recycled air and less fresh air are often used in an effort to save money.

Outdoor air pollution often comes in the form of automobile and industrial exhaust. Exposure to these can cause hidden mineral deficiencies, which may affect any and every organ.[19] Primarily affected is the respiratory system. Pulmonary irritation, asthma and chronic bronchitis are common symptoms of air pollution exposure.

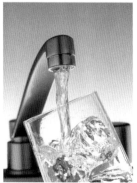

More than 700 chemicals have been identified in American drinking water.[20] These include asbestos, pesticides, heavy metals, nitrates and a variety of chemicals, including those known to be carcinogenic.[21] Two of the most damaging substances, both to over-all health and to digestive function, found abundantly in the water supply are chlorine and fluoride.

The late Dr. John Yiamouyiannis, author of *Fluoride the Aging Factor*, stated that fluoride interferes with enzyme activity and the body's use of oxygen. Fluoride poisoning can result in nausea and vomiting, constipation, loss of appetite, sores in the mouth and on the lips, weight loss, discoloration of teeth, skin rash, increased salivation, shallow breathing, stomach cramps and pain, bloody vomit and many other symptoms throughout the body.

Chlorine, added as a disinfectant to water, becomes a problem when it unites with other pollutants and/or organic matter, such as decaying vegetation, to form trihalomethanes (ThMs). These chemical compounds include such deadly chemicals as chloroform, bromoform and carbon tetrachloride and have been linked with increased incidences of colon and rectal cancer as well as bladder cancer.[21]

Notes

[1] Melissa Palmer, MD, *Hepatitis and Liver Disease*, Avery Publishing Group, 2000, p. 377.

[2] William R. Kellas, Ph.D and Andrea Sharon Dworkin, ND, *Surviving the Toxic Crisis*, Professional Preference, 1996, p. 139.

[3] Ibid., p. 213.

[4] Ibid., p. 229.

[5] Jacqueline Krohn, MD and Frances Taylor, MA, *Natural Detoxification*, Hartley and Marks Publishers, Inc., 2000, p. 102.

[6] Op. Cit., Kellas and Dworkin, p. 7.

[7] Susan Stockton, *The Terrain is Everything*, Power of One Publishing, 2000, p. 123.

[8] Ibid., p. 122.

[9] Ibid., p. 123.

[10] Op. Cit., Kellas and Dworkin, p. 52.

[11] Ibid., p. 73.

[12] Ibid., p. 159.

[13] Ibid., p. 59.

[14] Ibid., p. 189.

[15] Ibid., p. 5.

[16] Op. Cit., Stockton, p. 127.

[17] Ibid.[18] Op. Cit., Krohn, p. 93.

[18] Op. Cit., Kellas and Dworkin, p. 89.

[19] Op. Cit., Stockton, p. 184.

[20] Ibid.

[21] Ibid., p. 185.

4

Chapter Summary

In addition to toxins generated from impaired digestion, the body is confronted with toxins from drugs, focal infection in the oral cavity and a wide array of environmental toxins. These include electromagnetic pollution from 60-cycle current, as well as the widespread use of microwave technology. Food additives and pesticides constitute a major source of chemical exposure. The body is further burdened by toxic metals abundant in the environment and even present in our teeth in the form of 'silver' fillings. Air and water pollution exposes us to such toxic elements as fluorine and chlorine.

> **Fluoride is more poisonous than lead and slightly less poisonous than arsenic.**
>
> **Drs. William R. Kellas and Andrea Sharon Dworkin,**
> *Surviving the Toxic Crisis*

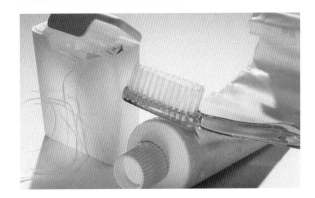

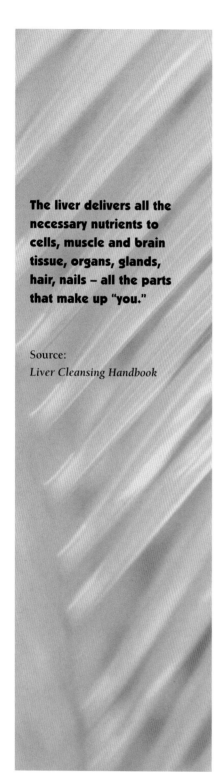

The liver delivers all the necessary nutrients to cells, muscle and brain tissue, organs, glands, hair, nails – all the parts that make up "you."

Source:
Liver Cleansing Handbook

CHAPTER 5

THE liver

The word 'liver' comes from the old English word for 'life.' The length and quality of life depends on how well the liver functions. The liver is the largest and most active internal organ. It is also the most over-worked and least cared for organ. A properly functioning liver:

- Manufactures 13,000 different chemicals
- Maintains 2,000 internal enzyme systems
- Filters 100 gallons of blood daily
- Produces 1 quart of bile daily

The typical 4-pound liver performs more than 500 unique bodily functions that are critical to life and well being. Six are primary functions:

- Manufactures bile for the emulsion of fat for digestion
- Makes and breaks down hormones, including cholesterol, testosterone and estrogen
- Controls regulation of blood sugar
- Filters all food, nutrients, drugs, alcohol and materials in the blood
- Detoxifies all endotoxins (internally produced) and exotoxins (environmental)
- Contains part of the immune system (Kuppfer cells) – They alert the body to the presence of pathogenic microbes and other toxins

Today, your liver has totally different issues with which to deal than did your grandmother's liver. Environmental pollution, prescription drugs, chemical food additives, water chlorination, household chemicals, pesticides and certain bacteria and fungi are relatively new toxins that impact our lives – and our livers – daily. We abuse our livers almost continuously, causing chronic fatigue, high blood pressure, elevated cholesterol levels, irritable bowel syndrome, brain fog, chronic indigestion or any number of other problems. In many cases, the

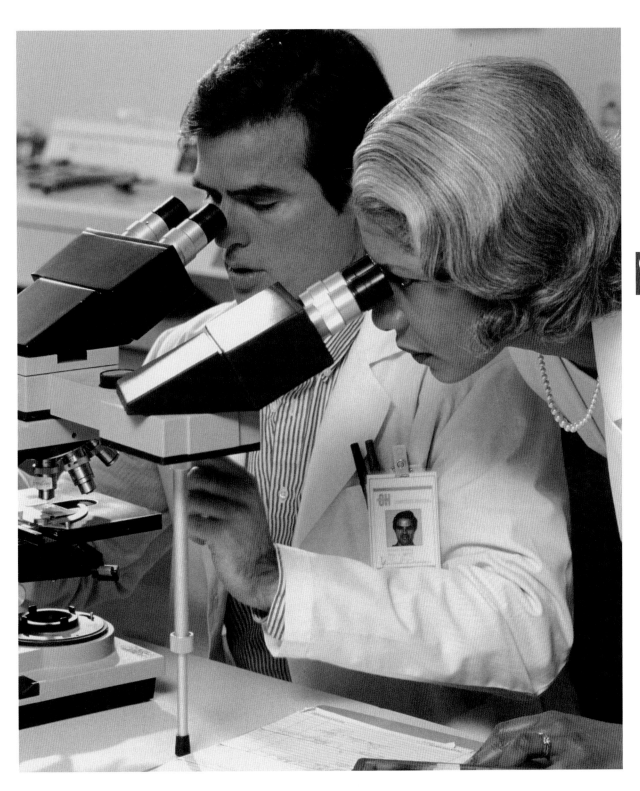

5

> **We live on fast foods, consume too much alcohol, abuse prescription drugs and live in a polluted world. In between too much coffee and soft drinks, we occasionally drink a bottle of designer spring water.**

typical response to these symptoms is to take drugs that further limit the liver's ability to function.

> **The liver can lose as much as 70% of its capability before liver disease is commonly diagnosed.**

Why do we not associate many health problems with the breakdown of the liver? Part of the reason is that liver dysfunction does not occur overnight.

With *functional* testing of the liver (feeding the person chemicals that require the liver to work and measuring the resultant by-products), early detection of liver problems is possible. Such testing has demonstrated that only one half of supposedly healthy test subjects had normal liver function! Asymptomatic liver dysfunction is thought to be a major cause of accelerated aging. As the liver becomes overwhelmed with internal and external toxins, other organs and systems can also become overloaded with toxins. These toxins will affect those areas of the body that are genetically weak. For example, if the immune system is inherently weak, an overload of toxins may result in chronic fatigue or allergies. In this instance, the causative role of the liver may not be recognized.

While the liver plays a key role in most metabolic processes, one of its primary functions is to manage the detoxification process. It is one of the

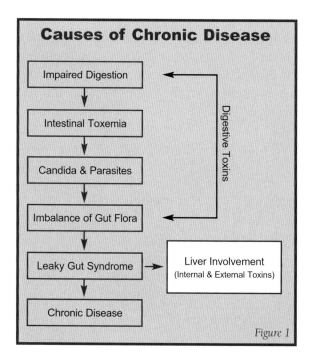

Figure 1

major organs of elimination in the body, along with the colon, kidneys, skin and lungs. Toxins in the liver are secreted largely in a water-soluble form into the blood to be excreted through the kidneys, and into the bile, to be eliminated by the colon. If the toxic load is great, the toxins can return to the liver from unfiltered blood in the kidneys and reabsorption of toxins from the intestines.

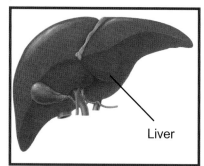

The liver is largely dependent upon the smooth operation of the digestive and eliminative organs. When the intestinal lining becomes too porous (leaky gut), toxins are rapidly absorbed, and the workload of the liver is increased. In addition, when the lungs, skin, kidneys and even the cells of the body are not correctly processing and eliminating toxins, there will be additional workload and stress on the liver. When the liver is overloaded, a domino effect is created, spreading toxicity throughout the system.

BILE SECRETION FOR FAT DIGESTION AND TOXIN ELIMINATION

Bile secretion is one of the liver's most important functions. Every day it manufactures approximately one quart of bile. Bile consists of bile salts, bilirubin, cholesterol, lecithin, hormones and electrolyes. In addition, it will contain toxins that have been processed by chemical reactions to render them safer for elimination. The bile is stored temporarily in the gallbladder, where water and minerals are reabsorbed, making the bile more concentrated, which improves its efficiency in digesting fat. In addition to emulsifying fat, bile helps lubricate the intestines and gives the stool its characteristic brown color. Where there is insufficient bile, the stool is light in color. Bile is released from the gallbladder and the liver as needed in response to the presence of fat in the intestines. In the gallbladder, the bile becomes a darker color. Good quality bile (reflected in a walnut brown stool) is important to good health. Not only does bile break down fat, but it also

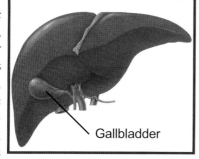

Gallbladder

assists in absorption of fat-soluble vitamins and in the assimilation of calcium. Additionally, it converts beta-carotene into vitamin A and promotes peristalsis, helping food residue move through the intestines and preventing constipation.

Bile serves as a carrier medium for the elimination of many toxic substances from the body. The bile and the toxins it carries are absorbed by dietary fiber in the intestines and excreted. In the absence of sufficient dietary fiber, the toxins (and the bile) are reabsorbed. Even more damaging than the reabsorption is the alteration of these toxins that often occurs when they interact with bacteria in the intestine.

Since bile is the carrier medium for the elimination of toxins from the body, diminished bile flow (cholestasis) is a significant contributor to liver impairment. When excretion of bile is inhibited, toxins remain in the liver too long. The liver can store these toxins (especially the fat-soluble ones) in its fatty tissue. As the liver stores more toxins, its efficiency is compromised, and bile flow decreases. **The liver can become constipated just like the colon.** Another problem can occur when bile ducts become blocked, usually by gallstones. Gallstone formation is thought to be due to an imbalance of bile salts and minerals, dehydration, toxins and excess cholesterol in the bile. In addition, a high fat, low fiber diet and pregnancy have been associated with gallstone production. Gallstones can be a real medical problem, blocking the flow of bile from the liver and gallbladder, and sometimes obstructing the pancreas and intestines as well. These

Functions of Cholesterol

- Essential for cell wall construction
- A building block for sex and adrenal hormones
- Needed for vitamin D synthesis
- Needed for production of bile salts
- Needed for proper functioning of the nervous system
- An antioxidant

Figure 2

5

situations often constitute a surgical emergency. In less urgent cases, small gallstones often can be dissolved medically with a special acid that is a natural product of the body. Yet another common problem is the excretion of toxic bile (bile that has not been chemically transformed adequately by the liver's enzyme system). Toxic bile can literally burn the bile ducts, the gallbladder and the intestines, eventually leading to hepatitis, cholecystitis, pancreatitis, and duodenitis (inflammation of the liver, gallbladder, pancreas and duodenum). Toxic bile could ultimately contribute to the development of cancer of the involved organs. An early sign of toxic bile is recurrent pain in these organs in the right upper abdomen.

Gallbladder problems then can develop when the liver is so overloaded that it sends toxins on to the gallbladder or duodenum before they are fully neutralized. Irritation from these toxins can cause the gallbladder to malfunction and irritate the pancreas and duodenum causing inflammation.

HORMONE REGULATION

The liver metabolizes hormones, notably testosterone and estrogen. The nutrient status of the individual will largely determine if estrogen is properly metabolized or becomes excessive in the body. Poor liver function, coupled with a deficiency of 'good' colonic bacteria, results in hormonal imbalances in both men and women that can put them at risk for developing serious disease.

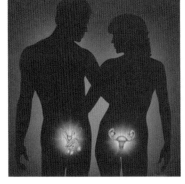

Certain B vitamins are needed by the liver to detoxify estrogen and excrete it in the bile.[1] With today's widespread vitamin B deficiencies, estrogen is not metabolized properly, and the result is increased levels of toxic estrogen metabolites. Excessive estrogen plus toxic metabolites produce cholestasis (diminished bile flow), resulting in further reduction in estrogen detoxification and clearance. **Conditions such as PMS, fibrocystic breast disease, ovarian cysts, uterine fibroids and cancer of the breast, ovaries and uterus have been associated with elevated estrogen.**

Cholesterol, a 'fat-like steroid alcohol,' and its contribution to heart disease is widely misunderstood. It is a substance found in all animal fat, and it serves many vital functions, as indicated in figure 2.

> **Although some cholesterol is absorbed from food, the bulk of it is manufactured in the liver. The liver not only synthesizes cholesterol, it is also critical in controlling cholesterol levels in the blood.**

The condition of the liver is actually far more important in determining cholesterol level than is the amount of animal fat consumed. If the liver is functioning optimally, and if the animal products consumed are of the highest quality (from grass-fed animals, raised organically) and man-made fats (hydrogenated) are avoided, the risk of heart disease from dietary causes should be minimal.

A healthy liver converts dietary cholesterol into bile and temporarily slows its own production. Bile is reabsorbed in direct proportion to the amount of time it takes to pass from the digestive tract. Where there is slow transit time through the digestive tract (as with constipation), there is excessive reabsorption of bile, as well as the toxins in the bile. This will decrease the ability of the liver to function properly.

BLOOD SUGAR REGULATION

The liver's energy production function is directly related to the creation of **glucose tolerance factor (GTF)** from the mineral chromium and the amino acid glutathione. GTF and insulin regulate blood sugar levels. The liver works with the pancreas and adrenal glands to regulate blood sugar. If too much sugar comes quickly to the liver from the intestinal tract, the liver will rapidly convert part of the sugar to **triglycerides** (fats), some of which is stored and some released into the blood to be reconverted into **glucose** (blood sugar) inside the cells. This process is extremely important, as it is the primary manner in which dietary sugar can be slowly released into the blood. Elevated blood sugar will cause serious problems. First, the sugar literally sticks to the blood proteins, which can cause the immune system not to recognize the sugar-coated proteins, and an immune attack can occur, which results in free radical production and cellular damage. Second, higher than average blood sugar levels will cause a chronic overproduction of insulin. This desensitizes the cellular insulin receptors, so that the sugar does not enter the cells efficiently, keeping the blood sugar high, creating a vicious cycle leading to type II diabetes. Finally, chronically elevated insulin levels greatly contribute to fat storage and increased production of cholesterol by the liver. It is obvious that the liver is important in controlling blood sugar levels. In addition, the liver stores sugars not required for immediate energy production. When stored, these sugars are known as '**glycogen**.' The liver also reconverts glycogen into glucose, which is fuel for the cells, when needed for energy.

THE PROCESSING OF ALL MATERIALS IN THE BLOOD

A major function of the liver is to filter blood, neutralizing and removing toxins and other harmful substances. Blood moves from the intestinal tract through the **portal vein** to the liver. Poisons from the intestines, including heavy metals, are typically deactivated in the liver.

Some of what is filtered is chemically neutralized and exported from the body through bile or through the kidneys. Many of the toxins, however, are chemically changed into a more active form and 'tagged' for recognition, so they can later be neutralized and eliminated from the body.

> **Approximately two quarts of blood pass through the liver every minute for detoxification.**

As long as our filter, the liver, stays clean, it can quickly break down such toxins as coffee, alcohol, nicotine, drugs, pesticides and food additives. A properly functioning liver is able to clear 99% of toxins from the blood before they enter the general circulation. Because of the liver's central role in detoxification, the major difference between a person who experiences symptoms when exposed to toxins and one who does not is in the ability of his/her liver to detoxify the blood adequately.

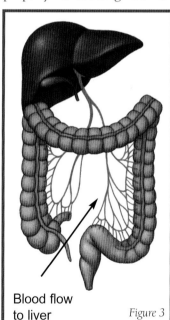

Blood flow to liver

Figure 3

THE DETOXIFICATION PROCESS

Detoxification is the process of filtering and removing toxins from the body. The body can eliminate toxins by either:

• **Excreting them directly** via the kidneys, colon, skin and lungs

OR

• **Chemically converting them** into substances that can be excreted by the liver into the bile or, if necessary, stored in the body

There are basically *two* types of toxins. Toxins that enter the body from the environment are called exotoxins. Some examples are prescription drugs, alcohol, pesticides, heavy metals and food additives. Anything that enters the body and cannot become food for cells probably needs to be filtered and eliminated. Toxins are also created inside the body. These internally generated toxins are called endotoxins. Endotoxins often originate in the intestinal tract. Many endotoxins are created from undigested food or as a by-product of the overgrowth of bacteria or fungi. Undigested food, acted on by certain types of bacteria, 'putrefies,' producing ammonia or alcohol. Such bacteria can produce many different toxins like ammonia, indol or skatole. Regardless of the origin of these toxins, it is the function of the liver to process and filter them. The toxins should then be excreted in the kidneys or colon.

Phase I and Phase II Detoxification

The liver's function is to transform fat-soluble chemicals into water-soluble compounds so they can be released through the kidneys and bowels. This transformation is carried out by a complex system of enzymes that are made in liver cells.

Phase I of detoxification involves activation of a series of enzymes with the technical name **cytochrome P450** mixed function oxidases, or cytochrome P450 for short. The cytochrome P450 system consists of 50 to 100 enzymes, each specializing in detoxification of certain types of chemicals. These enzymes metabolize or chemically break down toxins absorbed from the intestinal

---

In metabolizing a toxin, cytochrome P450 enzymes will do one of three things:

1. Transform the toxin to a less toxic form (neutralize it).
2. Make it water-soluble (so the kidneys can excrete it in the urine).
3. Convert it to a more chemically active form.

---

tract, hormones, alcohol, nicotine, drugs and a wide variety of chemicals from food and water. When the body is deficient in some of these enzymes its Phase I detoxification capability is limited.

Cytochrome P450 enzymes begin the transformation of toxins into non-toxic substances that can be excreted from the body. Many fat-soluble toxins must be converted into new substances called **active intermediaries**. These molecular intermediaries are often even more toxic than the original substances and therefore can do significant damage (especially by producing free radicals) if they're not promptly eliminated.

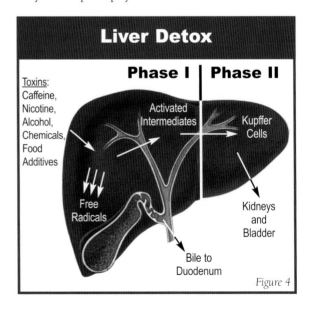

Liver Detox

Phase I | Phase II

Toxins:
Caffeine,
Nicotine,
Alcohol,
Chemicals,
Food
Additives

Activated Intermediates

Kupffer Cells

Free Radicals

Kidneys and Bladder

Bile to Duodenum

Figure 4

To function properly, cytochrome P450 requires specific nutrients: copper, magnesium, zinc and vitamin C. Research has shown that some substances activate P450, while others deactivate it. A sufficient intake of cabbage, broccoli and Brussels sprouts, as well as foods rich in B vitamins (whole grains) and vitamin C (peppers, tomatoes and citrus – excluding grapefruits and grapefruit juice) will ensure that the Phase I enzyme system is working well. Grapefruit, because it inhibits cytochrome P450, should not be eaten if toxic exposure is high or if drugs are being taken. The Phase I detox process tends to slow as we age.

If Phase I detoxification is inhibited, many prescription and over-the-counter drugs, caffeine, histamine, hormones, benzopyrene (from charbroiled meat), yellow dyes, carbon tetrachloride and insecticides will not be adequately detoxified and will instead be stored in the liver.

In Phase II, the intermediates must be converted a second time, combining with mineral compounds, amino acids or other biochemicals that are water-soluble and can be excreted in the urine and bile. This process of synthesis is described as **conjugation**. There are at least eleven of these conjugation processes in Phase II. Each process requires special nutrients and enzymes. If these processes are not functioning in the liver, then there is a delay in the breakdown of toxins, and they can build up in the body.

DYSFUNCTIONS

The liver is a strong and durable organ which is frequently overworked due to the enormous amount of toxicity in today's world. **As previously stated, the liver can continue to function when as much as 70% of its capacity is lost.** Many people today have livers that are functioning at only 25–30% of capacity – and many of these people are deluded into thinking that they are 'well.' In truth, they are accidents waiting to happen! Liver function can be as low as 20%, and we can still maintain life – and still not know for sure that we have liver problems.

A liver functioning at 20–30% of capacity may result in symptoms of poor health. These symptoms may be coming from seemingly unrelated organs and so not be recognized as liver-related. Many disease symptoms are the result of the liver losing its regulatory capability due to toxic overload, which is often a result of fermentation and

Causes of Phase II Liver Dysfunction

- We are ill, and our livers aren't functioning well.
- Toxic load is more than the liver can handle.
- Nutrients aren't available for detoxification.
- The digestive tract is overburdened with endotoxins, and conditions such as constipation and leaky gut develop.

Figure 5

Symptoms of Liver Problems

- Jaundice
- Pale stools
- Pain in the right side
- Depressed appetite
- Metallic taste in the mouth
- Loss of energy
- Frontal headaches
- Fatigue
- PMS
- Emotional excess
- Allergies
- Weak tendons, ligaments, muscles
- Chemical sensitivities
- Discoloration of the whites of the eyes
- Pain under the right shoulder blade
- Digestive complaints
- Poor tolerance to fatty foods
- Drowsiness after eating
- Constipation
- Skin problems

Figure 6

putrefaction in the intestines. A liver that is over-burdened with intestinal toxins is more vulnerable to the cumulative effects of environmental and other toxins.

The overloaded liver does not have the capability to detoxify adequately. Toxins then circulate to all parts of the body where they're retained. When symptoms of liver problems occur, they may include those listed in figure 6. These symptoms can be signs of a 'congested' or 'sluggish' liver. Then again, there may be no symptoms of liver dysfunction until a vast percentage of liver function is lost.

Liver function is impaired by many factors, including stress, drugs, alcohol, the accumulation of toxins from poor digestion and oral foci, the presence of fungi and parasites, inadequate nutrition, low thyroid function (hypothyroidism), smoking, environmental pollution and negative emotions.

Among the more serious liver problems are hepatitis and cirrhosis.

> **John Matsen, ND stated that liver overload may be the unsuspected cause of varicose veins and hemorrhoids:**
>
> *In the same way that the intestinal blood flows to the liver, so does the blood in the veins. If the liver is overloaded, then the blood in the veins tends to back up, causing increased pressure on the walls of the veins. If this increased pressure is combined with weakened vein walls due to poor mineral and/or vitamin absorption, the walls may dilate.*[2]

Hepatitis

Hepatitis is inflammation of the liver. It can be acute or chronic, depending upon the time it has lasted. Chronic hepatitis, which lasts longer than six months, may result in a more serious liver problem, cirrhosis (discussed below). Those with chronic hepatitis typically have few, if any, symptoms. Acute hepatitis may produce extreme symptoms in one individual, while causing only flu-like symptoms in another. Symptoms may include jaundice, fever, decreased appetite, abdominal pain, nausea, vomiting and fatigue. Typically, the urine is dark and the stools light.

Hepatitis is most often caused by viruses (A, B, C or D). It can, however, also result from autoimmune liver disease, obesity, alcohol and some medications.

Cirrhosis

Cirrhosis, which can result from alcoholism, a virus or some other chronic disease, involves permanent destruction of liver cells and irreversible scarring. The liver becomes hard and lumpy. Cirrhosis is an end product of a number of different liver diseases. Some people with cirrhosis have difficulty forming blood clots; some may develop **edema** (water retention) as a result of the extra load on the kidneys. **Osteoporosis** (decreased bone mass) is another potential complication of cirrhosis. People with cirrhosis of the liver tend to have a higher incidence of liver cancer and other cancers as compared with the general population.

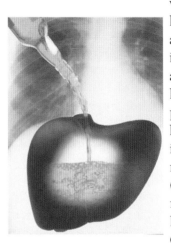

As serious as cirrhosis is, this disease, like other liver diseases, may be largely 'silent' for many, meaning that it may produce only vague symptoms: fatigue, loss of appetite, nausea and decreased libido.

The jaundice associated with hepatitis may also be present with cirrhosis. It is caused by elevation of **bilirubin**, the yellow pigment that the liver produces when it recycles worn out blood cells.

Both hepatitis and cirrhosis can be the net result of an overburdened liver unable to perform adequately its detoxification functions.

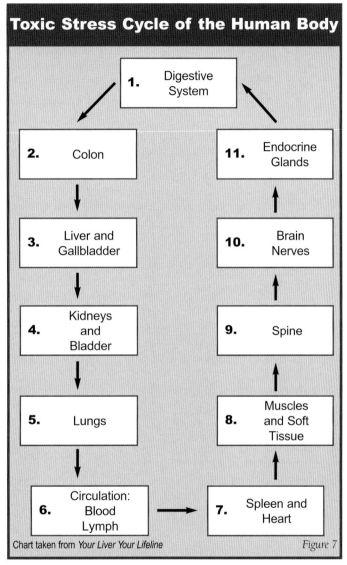

Toxic Stress Cycle of the Human Body

1. Digestive System
2. Colon
11. Endocrine Glands
3. Liver and Gallbladder
10. Brain Nerves
4. Kidneys and Bladder
9. Spine
5. Lungs
8. Muscles and Soft Tissue
6. Circulation: Blood Lymph
7. Spleen and Heart

Chart taken from *Your Liver Your Lifeline*   *Figure 7*

degeneration sets in (figure 7).

The digestive system is the starting point in the toxic stress cycle. When food is not properly digested, toxins are produced in the bowel. These toxins then travel to the liver via the portal vein. The liver, stressed and congested from toxic overload (and nutrient deficiency), is incapable of managing the toxins and so passes them through the hepatic veins into the systemic circulation. A portion of the toxins may be secreted through the skin, kidneys and lungs as the toxin-laden blood reaches these organs. The remainder of the toxins are stored in the bones, hair, muscles (both skeletal and heart muscle), lymphatic tissue or the fat. These toxins greatly affect energy production and hormone and enzyme function that controls free radical production. When these cellular functions are impaired, the body suffers and gradually becomes diseased.

Since the toxic stress cycle begins with poor digestion, which sends toxins to the colon and then to the liver, the key to interrupting this cycle is the simultaneous support of these key organs:

Toxic Stress Cycle

When the liver is overburdened with toxins and thus limited in its capability to neutralize them, some are stored and some are recycled. This recycling of toxins has been termed the 'toxic stress cycle.' The late master herbalist, Stuart Wheelwright, taught about this key process in disease causation. The toxic stress cycle begins when an overload of toxins is passed from organ to organ in the body until either detoxification occurs or

- Liver
- Intestines (small and large)
- Stomach

Because the self-perpetuating toxic stress cycle is set in motion largely through improper eating habits, a proper diet helps to stop it. Chapter 10 has details on improving digestion (and thus liver function) through diet.

Liver Function Tests

To evaluate the ability of the liver to detoxify, practitioners of what has been called 'functional medicine' (a term coined by Dr. Jeffrey Bland) use special functional testing. One such test involves having the patient swallow capsules containing caffeine, which is detoxified primarily by cytochrome P450 (in Phase I). Phase I detox capability is evaluated on the basis of how quickly the caffeine disappears from the blood or saliva. If it does so very slowly, detoxification by the patient is considered poor, owing to low cytochrome P450 activity. If the caffeine disappears rapidly, then the patient has a higher detoxification rate of cytochrome P450 activity. Genetics, degree of toxic exposure and nutritional status are all factors that account for individual differences in Phase I detox capacity and therefore differences in susceptibility to various diseases. Someone whose cytochrome P450 system is functioning well can take much more toxic abuse than one whose P450 system is not working well.

> **Research has shown that specific foods and nutrients not only have a beneficial effect on detoxification capability, but can also provide a safe and viable approach to treating a variety of immune disorders and toxicity syndromes.**

> **While sophisticated laboratory tests are necessary to prove a dysfunction of a specific liver detoxification system, several signs and symptoms can give us a good idea of when our liver's detoxification systems are not functioning well or are overloaded. In general, any time you have a bad reaction to a drug or environmental toxin, you can be pretty sure there is a detoxification problem.**
>
> **Michael Murray, N.D. and**
> **Joseph Pizzorno, N.D.,**
> ***Encyclopedia of Natural Medicine***

Another test involves swallowing a capsule of acetaminophen (Tylenol), which is detoxified primarily by Phase II detox reactions. Once detoxified, it is excreted through the urine, which is then sent to a laboratory for analysis. The amount and type of substances found in the urine indicate the efficiency of the subject's Phase II detox systems.

A person with poor Phase II conjugation activity (indicated by presence of certain substances in the urine), but rapid Phase I detox capacity, is accumulating toxins that had been created by Phase I activity, though unable to effectively eliminate them from the body (due to low Phase II activity). The result is a build up of intermediary toxic substances, which can be the cause of many problems, as these can be more toxic than the original toxic substances.

The remedy for this situation is to lower the toxic load on the body and to balance Phase I/Phase II. This could translate into reduced use of alcohol and/or drugs. A wholesome diet must be adopted and appropriate nutrients supplemented to support Phase II conjugation. Sources of endotoxins (poor digestion and focal infection) must also be addressed.

People with very slow cytochrome P450 detox activity (Phase I) tend to be environmentally sensitive, with a history of allergy or asthma. Dr. Jeffrey Bland classifies people into one of three categories of detoxifiers based on the caffeine and acetaminophen tests described above. They are:

Fast Detoxifiers
They have rapid cytochrome P450 (Phase I) activity and rapid liver conjugation (Phase II) activities.

Slow Detoxifiers
They have slow cytochrome P450 activity (Phase 1) and slow liver conjugation (Phase II) activities.

Imbalanced Detoxifiers
They have rapid cytochrome P450 activity (Phase I) but depressed conjugation (Phase II) activities.

It is the third group that is most likely to experience health problems as a result of their impaired detox ability. This is due to an increase of intermediary toxins in their systems. These toxins can adversely affect the endocrine, immune and nervous systems.

Notes
[1] Michael Murray, ND and Joseph Pizzorno, ND, *Encyclopedia of Natural Medicine*, Prima Health, 1998, p. 736.

[2] John Matsen, ND, *The Mysterious Cause of Illness*, Fischer Publishing Corporation, 1987, p. 44.

Chapter Summary
The liver, among its many other functions, filters toxins out of the blood carried to it from the stomach, small intestine and colon. It manages these toxins through a 2-phase enzyme system through which toxins are made more water-soluble for excretion. Certain nutrients, particularly vitamins, minerals and amino acids, are required for these detox systems to function properly.

Those people most prone to chronic illness have rapid Phase I systems but depressed Phase II systems. This is because a build up of bio-transformed intermediaries from Phase I detoxification increases overall toxicity.

When the liver is overburdened with toxins, some are stored for later detoxification and elimination. Toxins may also be passed to other organs of elimination. If these back-up organs fail to neutralize them, toxins may be stored in fatty tissues of the body, leading ultimately to development of degenerative disease.

Besides the intestinal toxins produced through impaired digestion, the liver must manage other toxic stressors such as drugs, focal infection and environmental toxins (discussed in chapter 4).

In addition to its detoxification function, the liver also manufactures bile, makes and breaks down hormones, controls regulation of blood sugar and manufactures and regulates cholesterol.

5

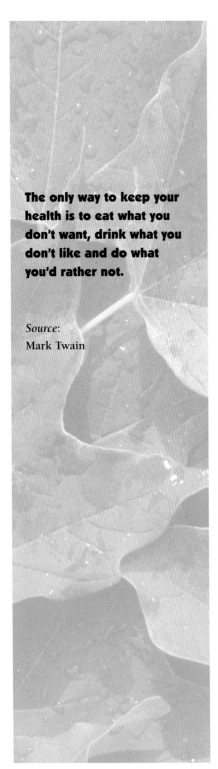

The only way to keep your health is to eat what you don't want, drink what you don't like and do what you'd rather not.

Source:
Mark Twain

CHAPTER 6

THE HEALING
process: MOVING INTO WELLNESS

This chapter presents guidelines to enhance the digestive process, the first step in the prevention of disease as aging occurs. Whether we experience minor symptoms like fatigue or heartburn or already have such conditions as fibromyalgia or irritable bowel syndrome, the process of healing and restoring the body to health involves taking certain steps. Maintaining good health requires wise choices. Health is not just the absence of disease or pain. Holistic health is defined in terms of the whole person, not in terms of diseased body parts. It encompasses the psychological, mental, emotional, social, spiritual and environmental aspects of the individual. Health is a continuum, with optimal health at one end, and toxic overload, which may manifest itself as cancer, autoimmune disease or some other form of disease or disability, at the opposite end. Optimal health is a dynamic process that is always moving in one direction or the other on this continuum (see figure 1).

A proactive approach is required to achieve optimal health regardless of where a person's health is located on the continuum. People who feel good are less likely to believe they need to take preventive measures such as cleansing (detoxification) programs or adding digestive enzymes to their diet. These are a must in today's world because no one is totally protected. People who are experiencing toxic overload (bottom of the continuum) are usually in pain. They often reach for a more holistic approach when modern medicine no longer seems to work. These people must begin to take responsibility and action if health is to be regained to any degree!

The process of restoring wellness to the body begins by creating a lifelong maintenance/prevention program. If people hold steadfast to this goal once health has been restored, then they will increase the chances of being free of pain and the need for medication.

As 'The Healing Process' (figure 2) indicates, managing stress and enhancing digestion are the first two steps toward vibrant health.

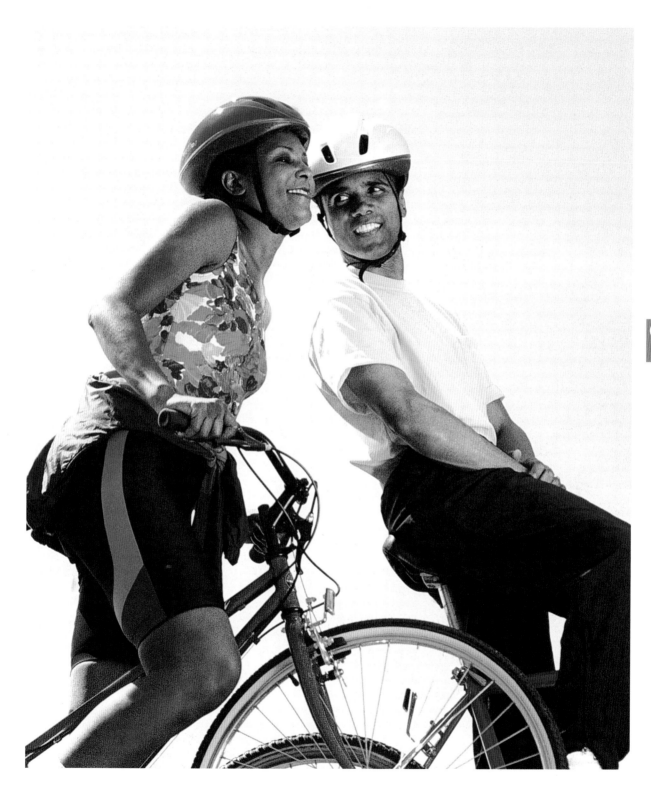

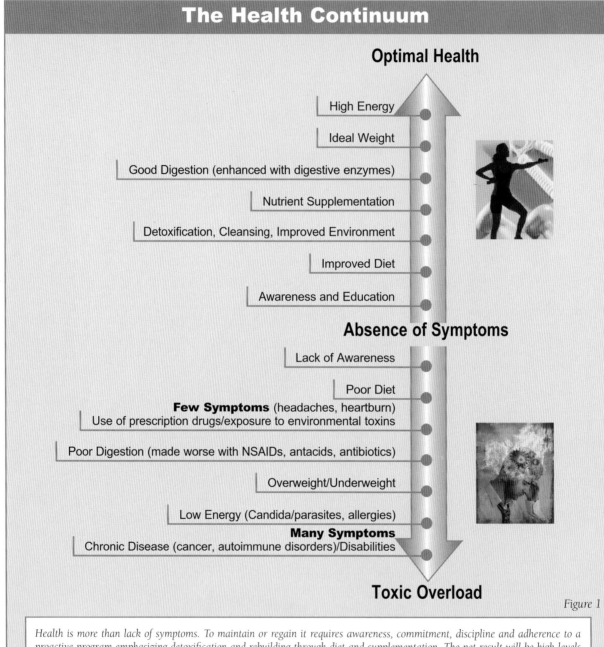

The Health Continuum

Optimal Health

High Energy

Ideal Weight

Good Digestion (enhanced with digestive enzymes)

Nutrient Supplementation

Detoxification, Cleansing, Improved Environment

Improved Diet

Awareness and Education

Absence of Symptoms

Lack of Awareness

Poor Diet

Few Symptoms (headaches, heartburn)
Use of prescription drugs/exposure to environmental toxins

Poor Digestion (made worse with NSAIDs, antacids, antibiotics)

Overweight/Underweight

Low Energy (Candida/parasites, allergies)

Many Symptoms
Chronic Disease (cancer, autoimmune disorders)/Disabilities

Toxic Overload

Figure 1

Health is more than lack of symptoms. To maintain or regain it requires awareness, commitment, discipline and adherence to a proactive program emphasizing detoxification and rebuilding through diet and supplementation. The net result will be high levels of energy and a sense of well-being.

The road to chronic disease and disability, on the other hand, begins with lack of awareness, poor diet and symptom suppression through use of pharmaceutical drugs. Here the stage is set for the development of digestive dysfunction, which increases the body's toxic load and depletes its energy. The net result is development of more and more symptoms, leading ultimately to degenerative disease.

MANAGE STRESS

The balance of mental, emotional and spiritual health in any individual is extremely important. Stress comes in many forms, and it is important to identify the source(s). Stress often stems from problems with relationships, work and/or finances.

How do you find relief from stressful situations that occur in life? It depends on your everyday choices. For example, after a stressful day at work, do you take a walk, or stop at a bar for a few drinks?

The digestive system, as noted, is very sensitive to stress levels. The capability of the organs to produce enzymes can be adversely affected by stress. As stress continues, there is a notable increase in intestinal permeability, which can allow for the absorption of undigested food. Chapter 2 dealt with food sensitivities, and how undigested food particles enter the bloodstream through the bowel wall (leading to an allergic response). The body reacts with antibody production against the undigested food because it is identified as 'foreign.' During *any*

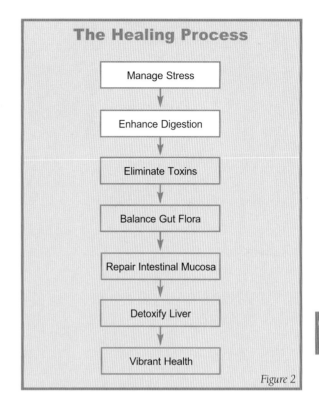

The Healing Process

Manage Stress → Enhance Digestion → Eliminate Toxins → Balance Gut Flora → Repair Intestinal Mucosa → Detoxify Liver → Vibrant Health

Figure 2

6

stress response, we go into sympathetic dominance, and digestion suffers, because blood and energy are diverted away from the digestive organs toward the skeletal muscles and brain – preparing the body for fight or flight. Eating should never occur when in such a state. If so, the food will not be digested, and an allergic reaction or sensitivity to it may well develop.

Regardless of degree of hunger, it is best to forgo eating until the stress response subsides or is consciously eliminated. Such conscious control can be learned by practicing techniques for relaxation of the body and mind. These techniques may involve the practice of meditation and/or relaxation exercises, physical exercises and deep breathing. Spending 'quiet time' alone, perhaps in a serene outdoor environment, may help reduce stress, as may listening to soothing music or recordings of nature sounds. Warm baths can be relaxing,

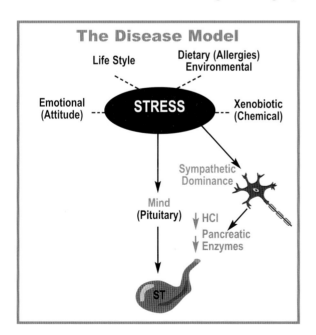

The Disease Model

Life Style

Dietary (Allergies) Environmental

Emotional (Attitude)

STRESS

Xenobiotic (Chemical)

Sympathetic Dominance

Mind (Pituitary)

↓ HCl

↓ Pancreatic Enzymes

ST

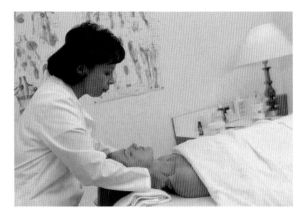

as can massages. The practice of 'giving thanks' and maintaining a moment of silence before eating is one that is certainly conducive to relaxation and thus to good digestion as well.

It has been discovered fairly recently that the bowel wall has a 'mind of its own,' so to speak, in that it actually contains the same receptors as the brain and undergoes similar neurological processes, especially with regard to serotonin receptors. Essentially then, the bowel quite literally makes 'decisions' with regard to absorption and motility. These decisions, like decisions made by the brain, can be hugely influenced by our emotional state.

There are additional steps to take to create a more harmonious lifestyle and relieve stress when the need arises. Important considerations in the management of stress are lifestyle factors such as time management and exercise.

Helpful time management practices include:

• Setting priorities – Be realistic in what can be accomplished.
• Creating a definite eating plan for the week
• Organizing the day

Exercise is of utmost importance in managing stress. As we exercise, we become stronger. The body functions more efficiently and develops greater endurance. Exercise also helps regulate blood sugar levels, so that energy is more sustained during the day. It helps the brain release **endorphins**, (morphine-like substances) that can lead to a euphoric or happy feeling. Exercise has been also shown to increase the blood levels of phenylethylamine, the chemical that is released when humans are in love! Exercise should be enjoyable, not a forced activity. Walking, yoga and biking, even though dissimilar activities, can all create the same sense of well being in a person and definitely help in creating better digestion, absorption and assimilation of nutrients from food.

ENHANCE DIGESTION

Enhanced digestion is the next step in the healing process. This requires:

• Following dietary guidelines
• Chewing foods thoroughly
• Eating consciously
• Eating a variety of foods
• Following food combining rules if digestion is compromised
• Supplementation with plant enzymes and HCl (hydrochloric acid) for better digestion

Following dietary guidelines certainly challenges most people in today's fast-paced environment, but it is decidedly the most critical component of healing and preventive health care.

There are many misunderstandings about food and nutrition. Even experts in the field of health can become confused: One day eggs are good; the next day they are reported to be bad. Fiber is good for lowering cholesterol and helping to prevent colon cancer, and then its benefits are questioned. Depending upon who's doing and reporting the research, there will always be conflicting findings.

The real challenge is finding the right balance. This comes with moderation and common sense. Excessive amounts of sugar and refined foods are very bad, not only for the digestive system, but also for the immune system. Diet is so important in creating good health that two chapters are devoted to it. Chapter 10 contains good preventive dietary information that can be useful to anyone. In it, we discuss the importance of whole foods and good fats and differentiate between healthy and unhealthy foods. Chapter 8 includes a detox diet, which is recommended for anyone suffering from Candida or any gastrointestinal problem or food sensitivity issue. This diet is meant to be used for a short period of time while the body is healing. Most foods to which people become sensitive are eliminated in this diet. While difficult to follow in the beginning, adherence to this diet for a period of time can result in vast improvements in health.

Thorough Chewing

Digestion begins in the mouth. If food is not chewed thoroughly, the amylase enzymes from the saliva aren't in contact with it long enough to begin the digestive process. When large bits of insufficiently chewed food move to the stomach, we may experience gas or indigestion. Eating too rapidly can cause bloating because excessive air is ingested. Many people chew their food only a couple of times before washing it down with water or some other beverage. This results in dilution of digestive juices and further digestive stress. Digestion can be improved by simply taking more time to thoroughly chew food, so that the first phase of carbohydrate digestion functions properly.

Eating on the run or making meal time social time, can divert attention from the eating (and chewing) process. If food is chewed less than 10 times before swallowing, then a concerted effort should be made to extend chewing time. Try chewing

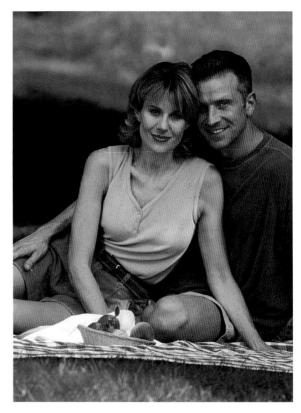

food as much as 30 times so that it is liquefied. The more thoroughly it is chewed, the better the digestive process will function.

Conscious eating is another important factor to ensure proper digestion of food. To support good digestion, the 'conscious' eater will want to:

• Prepare an enjoyable atmosphere for eating (not in the car).
• Eat in a relaxed atmosphere.
• Eat at a moderate pace. Slow down!

Cold liquids or excessive liquid intake should be avoided during meals. Cold beverages slow the digestive process. Too much liquid during meals dilutes enzymes, interrupting the digestive process. A small amount of room temperature liquid with meals (tea/water) is okay, as is taking supplements with water after meals.

6

Variety is the spice of life, and the body knows this instinctively. Eating the same foods again and again, day after day (especially processed foods), can increase food sensitivities. A rotation of foods, which reduces repetitive eating habits, is best.

Enzyme Supplementation

Historically, the best sources of enzymes have been from the consumption of fresh fruits and vegetables. Eating these foods on a daily basis is the foundation of good health. Even the food pyramid requires three to five servings of vegetables and two to three servings of fruit daily. Unfortunately, too many people disregard these daily guidelines.

Enzymes are essential for all chemical processes in the body, including digestion. The enzymatic level of fresh foods, such as fruits and vegetables, is reduced by long-term storage and pesticides and toxins in the water and soil. As we age, the number of enzymes and their activity levels decrease. This is why supplementation with enzymes is helpful.

Cooking food destroys enzymes, which are needed for virtually every chemical reaction in the body. For this reason, a diet that is at least 50% raw is recommended. However, we still have the problem of enzyme destruction with the 50% of the food that's cooked. The obvious solution is to

How Enzymes Break Down Foods

- Large food molecule
- Enzyme
- Smaller molecule
- Intestinal wall
- Blood vessel

Absorption

- Enzyme
- Tiny food molecule passes through intestine wall
- Molecule in blood vessel

Figure 3

use enzyme supplements. People with digestive problems will want to take digestive enzymes with every meal. Others may do so as well – or take them just with cooked meals.

A good enzyme supplement will not just substitute for the body in the digestive process: Supplementing with digestive enzymes will decrease the need for all of the pancreatic enzyme secretions to be active in the digestive tract. This will allow some of the pancreatic enzymes to be absorbed into the blood where they can work on that portion of food that enters the blood and lymphatic system undigested, helping to break it down. Pancreatic enzymes also enhance the immune system.

A good digestive enzyme formula will contain a variety of enzymes to address every type of food group ingested: fats, starches, dairy, plant, vegetable material (cellulose) and sugar. The ideal digestive enzyme supplement would be

Q. Will plant enzymes stop my digestive organs from producing their own enzymes?

A. No. Plant enzymes simply support your digestive process.

Fewer than 10 percent of Americans eat 2 servings of fruit or 3 servings of vegetables daily. Fifty percent eat no vegetables at all, 70 percent eat no vegetables or fruits rich in vitamin C, and 80 percent eat no vegetables or fruits rich in carotenoids per day.

plant-based. Such enzymes are already activated as they enter the system and therefore start to work in the stomach, continuing to function throughout the body with a broad pH range, from 2 to 14. When digestion is incomplete, plant enzymes act like 'Pac Man,™' breaking down and cleaning up undigested food in the digestive tract. This undigested food gives rise to toxin production in the intestinal tract, which would eventually lead to toxic overload.

Plant enzymes are the best choice for indigestion or as a preventive measure to ensure complete digestion. Anyone older than 40 should have plant enzymes in their daily regimen. It is also a good choice for people younger than 40, and for vegetarians. Plant enzymes can be taken at higher doses by people who have microbial infections (especially parasites) in the intestinal tract. These enzymes may be used by people with lower gastric distress: bloating, flatulence and cramping. Take one to three capsules with, or directly following, each meal. Refer to product inserts for information on specific products that match the profile above.

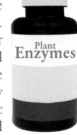

Plant Enzymes

People older than 40 who are deficient in HCl may address that deficiency by taking a HCl supplement. Those with Candida can also benefit from a HCl supplement, for they often have low levels of stomach acid. Those experiencing upper gastric distress – heartburn, reflux or belching – could benefit from taking products with HCl as well. HCl will prevent bacterial invasion by killing bacteria entering the mouth and stomach. A HCl-containing digestive formula is recommended while traveling to help prevent this invasion of bacteria.

Look for quality plant enzyme products that have high levels of protease and contain lipase, amylase, lactase, cellulase and invertase (for sugar). A good formula will also include ingredients like glutamine and gamma oryzanol to help support the lining of the digestive tract. A blend of herbs like ginger, marshmallow, bromelain and papaya should also be included in the formula. This type of enzyme mix is formulated for people who want to receive more nutritional value from the foods they eat.

6

If you are not sure you have low stomach acid, refer to the symptoms in Chapter 2. A stool test can also be done to detect the presence of undigested meat fibers. (See Resource Directory lab listing). HCl should be taken after a few bites of food (never on an empty stomach). If one capsule does not cause a warming sensation in the stomach, take another capsule with each meal until that sensation is experienced; when this occurs, one capsule less should be taken in the future. The amount of food eaten at a meal can also be a factor in how much HCl is needed. Once diet and health improve, less HCl is needed, and plant enzymes become the primary support for digestion.

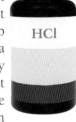

HCl

A good HCl supplement might also contain pepsin, quercitin, bromelain, butryric acid, N-acetyl-glucosamine, L-glutamine, gamma oryzanol and other soothing ingredients. See product inserts for more information on such a formula.

Some people with gastritis or heartburn can have *too much* stomach acid as a result of diet or stress. DGL (deglycyrrhizinated licorice) is a good choice for these people. Chewable DGL is taken before meals to soothe the stomach. It helps the cells of the stomach by improving the blood supply (and bringing nutrients to it). A good formula contains not only the DGL but also aloe and L-glutamine. Aloe is soothing to the mucosal lining, and L-glutamine helps restore this lining.

Those experiencing upper abdominal distress (heartburn, reflux or belching) may have an imbalance in their stomach. These symptoms can occur with too much acid, normal acid or even low acid in the stomach. Although this statement may appear contradictory, these different acid levels can cause the same symptoms. De-hydration can cause *any* amount of acid to irritate the stomach. When people do not drink enough water, 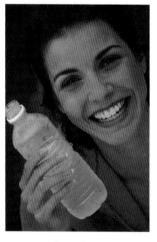 the mucous lining that is produced to protect the stomach from acid can be damaged and hampered in its ability to regenerate. A good rule of thumb is to drink a glass of room temperature water 30 minutes before a meal to protect and nourish the mucous lining so it can regenerate at regular intervals.

Acid irritation, combined with poor gastric digestion, can cause distention as well as reflux of food into the esophagus, which does not have the protective lining to deal with the acid. When such acid irritation occurs, HCl may be worth a trial because it can kill bacteria and help gastric protein digestion. This regimen, with the addition of digestive enzymes, aloe, DGL and glutamine, often completely relieves upper abdominal symptoms when combined with the right eating habits. It may be helpful, for a short period of time, to use acid blockers, but long-term use of antacids such as Pepcid, Zantac® and Prilosec® can create significant problems with digestion and microbial overgrowth, especially H. pylori, the bacterium that causes gastric and duodenal ulcers.

Chapter Summary

The healing process begins by identifying and managing stress in our lives and taking responsibility for finding healthy solutions. Developing time management skills and exercising regularly can do much to reduce stress levels.

The second step toward vibrant health is to enhance digestion. Digestive stress can be avoided by increasing intake of raw foods and through use of supplemental enzyme formulas with meals. Thorough chewing and eating in a relaxed environment are of utmost importance to digestion.

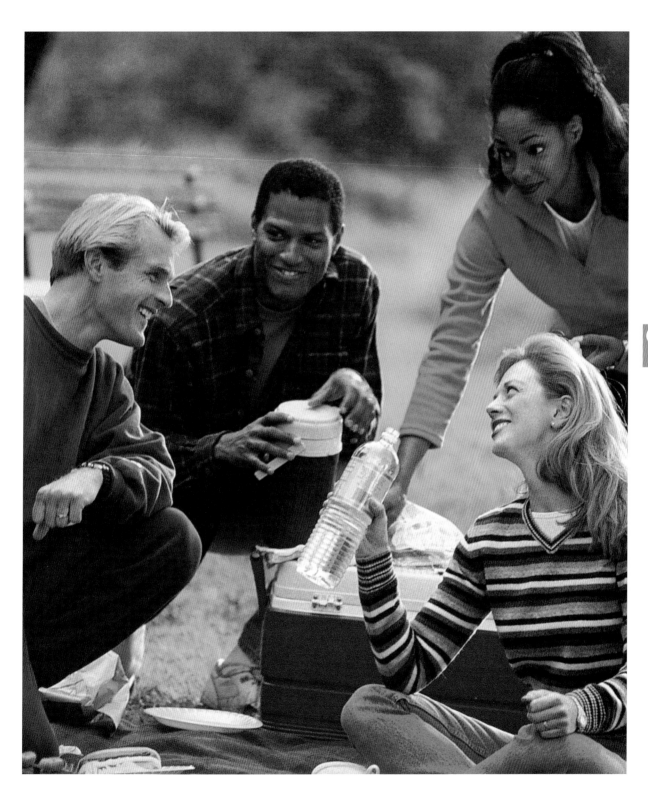

6

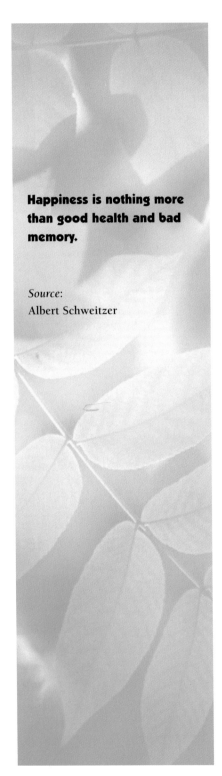

CHAPTER 7

ELIMINATION OF
toxins

Eliminating toxins is the third step on the road to digestive wellness and vibrant health. Cleansing and detoxification are essential to healing the digestive tract and restoring good liver function.

Detoxification is not a new concept. Many ancient cultures practiced detoxification in the form of fasting and colon cleansing with herbs. Toxins that are stored in the body can eventually overwhelm the liver. The result of this toxic overload is inflammation, which leads to chronic autoimmune disease. Toxins are foreign substances. The body will try to erect a barrier between these toxins and its own cells, organs and tissues. This barrier is inflammation, the body's attempt to protect itself from these toxic foreign substances. Inflammation can occur anywhere in the body where toxins are present. For example, if they are present in the joints, the result may be arthritis; if present in the colon, the result may be colitis. Toxic inflammation can be a direct cause of an almost endless list of chronic conditions. Even with diet improvements and a decrease in the impact of environmental toxins, the toxins that are stored in the body will remain there until removed. This is accomplished with detoxification and cleansing.

The Organs of Elimination

When asked, most people will define 'cleansing' as increased bowel elimination or just colon cleansing, and they think they will have to take a laxative, stay home from work and sit by the bathroom. Because toxins are present throughout the body, detoxification and cleansing cannot be limited to just bowel cleansing. Detoxification must be viewed as a total body process for all of the body's organ systems. These organ systems are collectively called the 'channels of elimination.' They must all be addressed if total body detoxification is to be effective. The five (5) primary channels of elimination are:

- Colon
- Kidneys

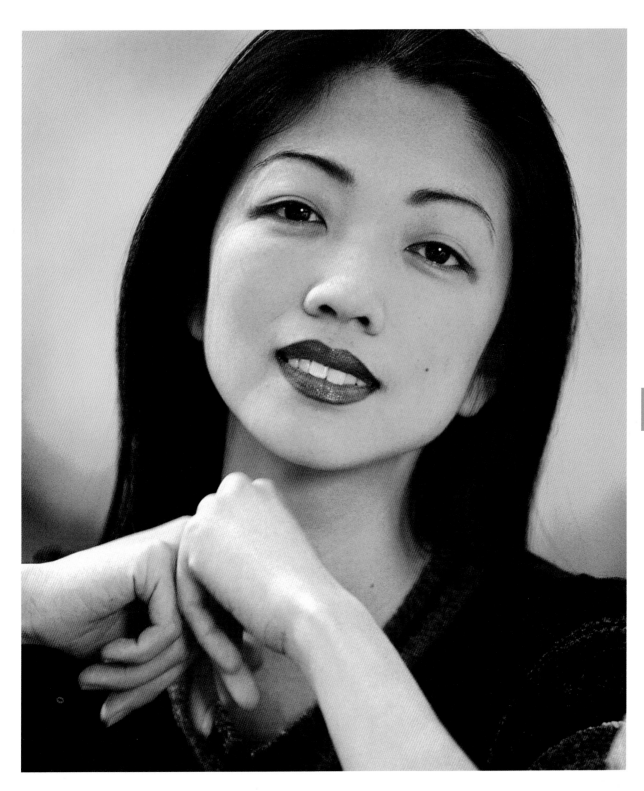

• Skin
• Lungs
• Liver

Colon cleansing is the very first step in the detoxification process. A clogged colon must be cleared first before embarking on any deeper cleansing programs (like Candida or parasites). Most people are unaware of having a colon that is clogged and backed up with toxic waste. Unfortunately, even if people have one elimination a day, they can still have considerable waste sitting in the colon creating toxins that can eventually lead to a chronic condition. By cleansing the colon first with herbs and colon hydrotherapy, a pathway is cleared for the rest of the organs to begin to detoxify.

In addition to the colon, kidneys, skin, lungs and liver, the blood (vascular system) and lymph (lymphatic system) are critical channels of elimination that must be supported for complete detoxification to occur. There are a number of approaches that can be used to facilitate cleansing and detoxification. Some of the most effective are:

• Dietary changes
• Herbal cleansing programs
• Colon hydrotherapy
• Saunas/steam baths/skin brushing
• Fasting
• Nutrient supplementation
• Exercise

It is important to note that most of these cleansing and detoxification methods have been successfully used to achieve and maintain health for thousands of years. Exercise, rather than an energetic lifestyle, is a relatively recent human activity.

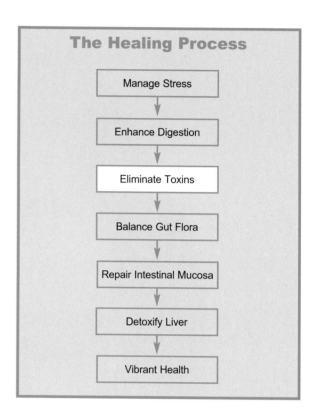

The Healing Process

Manage Stress

↓

Enhance Digestion

↓

Eliminate Toxins

↓

Balance Gut Flora

↓

Repair Intestinal Mucosa

↓

Detoxify Liver

↓

Vibrant Health

Diet

Adhering to dietary guidelines is a very important part of detoxification. Toxins cannot be cleared while they continue to enter the body. Chapter 10 presents a good general eating plan to be followed as a lifelong prevention program, and chapter 8 contains specifics of a diet for people with Candida, parasites and other conditions.

Drinking plenty of water during a cleanse is a necessity. The kidneys cannot perform adequately without sufficient water intake. The suggested amount is 1/2 ounce of water for every pound of body weight. It is important to drink the water in small amounts (about four ounces at a time) throughout the day, rather than guzzling a large amount at one sitting, to avoid straining the kidneys. Water, means *water*, and only water – not beverages containing water (especially not coffee, tea and soda, as they often contain caffeine, which

General Detox Guidelines
(Continue After Your Detox)

ELIMINATE	CHOOSE
Refined sugar	Honey, stevia or lo han
Caffeine, soda and alcohol	Water, herbal teas, green
Commercial salt (refined)	Use herbs/Celtic sea salt
Preservatives, artificial colors	Natural whole foods
Refined carbohydrates, white flour	Whole grains, organic
Pesticide-laden (commercial) foods	Organic vegetables and fruits
Artificial and refined oils	Cold pressed or unrefined oils
Processed meat	Meat free of antibiotics, hormones and drugs
Aspirin, Tylenol, antacids	White willow herb, plant enzymes

and distilled water. This may be accomplished by using a liquid supplement that is odorless, tasteless and colorless. Such liquid mineral supplements are available in local health food stores. Lyte Solution Concentrate, available through Health Equations (www.healtheqs.com, 1-800-328-2818), may be used for this purpose. One teaspoon of the liquid is added per gallon of purified water.

More toxins enter through the skin when bathing or showering than are ingested when drinking tap water. Therefore, some form of filtration in the shower or tub is necessary. A special zinc/copper 'KDF' medium is effective for this purpose.

Herbs

The use of herbs dates to the ancient Sumerians who described their medicinal use some 5,000 years ago. The first Chinese book of herbs was written in approximately 2700 BC. Most ancient cultures relied on herbs as their only medicine. The effects of herbs on the body are well known and documented. The *Herbal PDR* (Physician's Desk Reference), the *German Monagraph E* (a resource for physicians in Germany) and the National Institute of Health's (NIH) web site, www.NIH.org, all provide extensive information on many herbs.

> **Even today, almost 4 billion people (two thirds of the world's population) still rely on herbs as their primary medicine.**

has a dehydrating effect on the body.) During a cleanse, caffeine-containing beverages should be eliminated. If consumed at all after a cleanse, moderation is advised.

The issue of water *quality* is as important as the issue of quantity. As previously noted, pollution is widespread today – so widespread, that drinking untreated tap water can no longer be recommended. There are many types of water purification and filtration systems on the market today. The two most effective in removing pollutants are reverse osmosis (R/O) and distillation. Both methods remove all minerals along with pollutants, as there is no way to separate these. It is therefore necessary to return the minerals to R/O-treated

There are thousands of herbs with medicinal properties; however, only 25 or so are used regularly for cleansing and detoxification. There are basically two types of cleansing and detoxification herbs – those used for purification and those used for revitalization. **Purification herbs** are used to purge the organ systems. **Revitalizing herbs** help soothe and strengthen the organs.

Herbal Cleansing Programs

When it comes to herbal detoxification programs, you have two options: The first option is to have a customized program designed for you by a holistic physician.

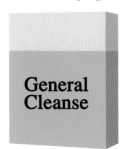

This might be necessary if you have moved into the 'many symptoms' area of the Health Continuum (chapter 6, figure 1). The alternative to a custom program would be a pre-formulated program. This alternative would be appropriate when detoxification is part of your prevention plan (as shown on the side of the continuum towards optimal health), or when your health has moved into the 'few symptoms' position.

When Candida and parasites are present, it is best to start with a general cleanse before using products designed to eliminate these organisms. The reason for this is that if parasites or yeast are killed, and the colon is dirty and the liver is toxic, you may have trouble eliminating these parasites quickly enough because the colon and liver are not functioning properly.

Since most of us in today's world lead busy, stressful lives, it is of utmost importance to keep the cleansing program as simple as possible. There are

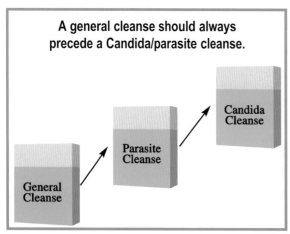

A general cleanse should always precede a Candida/parasite cleanse.

two areas to address in beginning a cleanse: The first focuses on the cleansing of the colon, while the second targets the remaining channels of elimination – liver, blood, lymph, skin, kidneys and lungs – supporting them with herbs. This is *whole body detoxification*.

When the liver is overburdened with toxins, the load is passed on through blood and lymph circulation to other organs of elimination: colon, kidneys, lungs and skin. It is therefore wise to begin a general cleanse that is designed to support all of these organs simultaneously, with special emphasis on the liver. General cleanse kits are easy to use and constitute a 30-day cleansing program. Such kits should include herbs that provide support for all organs and systems of elimination. Included in an effective herbal cleansing formula would be:

Milk thistle – stimulates bile secretion, acts as an antioxidant, and strengthens the cells of the liver to protect them.

Dandelion – stimulates bile and acts as a gentle laxative.

Beet – helps reduce damaging fats in the liver.

Artichoke leaf – stimulates secretion of bile and protects cells of the liver.

Mullein, an expectorant – helps expel mucus from the lungs.

Burdock – helps purge toxins that cause skin conditions.

Corn silk – a diuretic to flush the kidneys

Red clover – a blood purifier and expectorant

Larch gum – helps the lymphatic system.

The formula should also include herbs to support the heart (**hawthorne berry**) and the adrenal glands (**ashwaganda**). It must also address colon detoxification. Among other colon cleansing herbs, it would contain **aloe**, **rhubarb** and **triphala** to stimulate peristalsis and **magnesium hydroxide** to regulate water in the bowel. It is very important that the colon function properly or it will not be capable of eliminating toxins from the liver. These toxins will then recirculate, creating more of a problem. Formulas like this should be taken in the evening before retiring. Kits containing these herbs that address both colon and whole body cleansing make your cleanse very easy to perform.

Fiber is also important in a preventive or beginning detox program. Cleansing stimulates the liver to release toxins into the bile, which is then secreted back into the digestive tract (via the gallbladder). It is necessary to ingest extra fiber for these toxins to be absorbed and removed in the bowel elimination. One of the best fiber supplements is **flax**, as it is about 50% soluble and 50% insoluble fiber. **Soluble fiber** absorbs the toxins, and **insoluble fiber** sweeps the colon. Flax is also available in organic (pesticide-free) form, which is a plus. Never do a cleansing program without adding fiber for support to pick up and eliminate the toxins.

A final component in your complete body detox program would be daily intake of essential fatty acids from good quality oils. Essential fatty acids (EFAs) are fats the body cannot make from other materials and therefore must obtain from outside food sources. EFAs lubricate and soothe the colon. They are also crucial in virtually all vital functions of the body, including heart health and immunity. While there are several good sources of essential fatty acids, some of the best are:

1. **Fish oils** – high in Omega-3
2. **Flax** – high in vegetable Omega-3
3. **Borage** – high in Omega-9

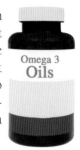

These essential oils are important in the digestive tract. A good product has the digestive enzyme lipase in the gel cap. Lipase is the enzyme that breaks down fat. It is a great way to enhance a detox program, for consuming oils without lipase puts a strain on the digestive organs.

Healing Crisis

While the net result of a cleanse will be elimination of toxins from the body, improved health and more energy, it is quite common to feel worse before feeling better. As herbal cleansing formulas kill disease-causing microorganisms such as Candida and parasites, toxins are released into the system. If they are released faster than the body can eliminate them, you may experience such symptoms as fever, fatigue, diarrhea, cramps, headache, increased thirst, loss of appetite, flu-like conditions, skin eruptions or irritations. These symptoms are due to a 'die-off' reaction known as the **Herxheimer Reaction** or **healing crisis**. It is sometimes difficult to distinguish between such a reaction and an actual illness. A natural health care practitioner can be of assistance in this regard. Generally speaking, the healing crisis is short-lived (a day or two, but usually no longer than a week). Symptoms may range from mild to severe, depending upon the rate of cleansing. The following steps will help to avoid, reduce or eliminate a severe healing crisis.

• Start at very low doses of your herbal cleansing formula – half the recommended dose (or less if necessary), and then gradually increase to the recommended level during a 30-day period.

7

• If liver support herbs are not present in your cleansing formula or you have a history of liver problems, support the liver with an appropriate herbal formula.

• Initiate the necessary dietary modification two weeks before starting the herbal cleanse.

• Get colon hydrotherapy sessions.

• Increase your water intake.

• Always take a fiber supplement.

A healing crisis, while uncomfortable to experience, is actually a sign of healing in progress. So if the symptoms are mild and tolerable, there is no need to adjust the dosage of your herbal cleansing product. Try to resist the temptation to suppress symptoms with drugs: it will only increase the body's toxic load and halt the cleansing process.

Saunas/Steam Baths

The skin is our largest organ, eliminating waste via perspiration. Heat causes toxins to be released from cells into the lymphatic fluid. Since sweat is manufactured from lymphatic fluid, the toxins from the lymph are released when the body perspires. Sweating occurs naturally during strenuous activity such as exercise; exposure to the sun; or being in a warm room. Saunas (dry heat) or steam baths (wet heat) create sweat intentionally for therapeutic purposes. This 'sweat (**hyperthermic**) therapy' not only releases toxins from the skin but also relaxes muscles, easing aches and pains. Releasing toxins via the skin through perspiration removes the load from the kidneys and liver, so those with impaired liver or kidney function may safely detoxify in this manner.

Raising the core temperature of the body through the hyperthermic effect has been shown to have a favorable impact upon the immune system. It is one of the few known ways to stimulate increased production of growth hormone, which helps the body shed fat, while maintaining lean muscle mass. Hyperthermic therapy also helps to restore autonomic nervous system function. This system

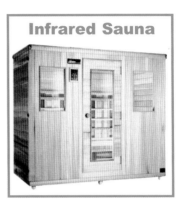

Infrared Sauna

governs muscle tension, sweating, blood pressure, digestion and balance. The autonomic nervous system is often dysfunctional in people with chronic fatigue and fibromyalgia. For this reason, people with these conditions can benefit from the two types of sauna therapies:

• Conventional sauna

• Infrared sauna

A conventional sauna heats the air either electrically or by the burning of wood. The skin perspires as a result of direct contact with the hot air. Typically, temperatures of 180 to 235 degrees Fahrenheit are used to induce sweating. These high temperatures increase cardiac load in the same way that aerobic exercise does.

Hal Huggins, DDS, an authority on mercury detoxification, recommends use of the sauna for detoxification. He suggests that the ill environmentally sensitive patient start out at a temperature of 135 degrees and work up to staying in the sauna for 45 minutes without discomfort, then leave the sauna at any sign of discomfort. Once 135 degrees is comfortably tolerated for 45 minutes, temperature may be gradually increased to 145 degrees.[1] (These temperatures apply to a conventional sauna, not infrared.)

In recent years, infrared saunas have been widely used for their superior therapeutic effect. Infrared heat is radiant heat. It heats objects directly without heating the air in between. In the infrared sauna, only 20% of the infrared energy heats the air; the other 80% is directly converted to heat within the body. The result is that the body perspires more quickly at lower temperatures than in a conventional sauna. The heat also penetrates more deeply, although without the discomfort and draining effect often experienced in a conventionally heated sauna. An infrared sauna produces two to three times more sweat volume, and because of the lower temperatures used (110-130 degrees), it is considered safer for those at cardiovascular risk.

Infrared saunas have been successfully used by people suffering from sports injuries, arthritis, chronic fatigue and fibromyalgia as well as other painful conditions. These saunas accelerate the removal of toxic metals as well as organic toxins like PCBs and pesticide residues – chemicals that

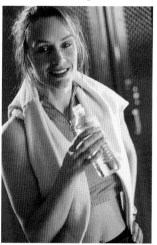

are stored in the fatty tissues of the body and are not easily dislodged. The heat produced in infrared saunas is extremely beneficial for those suffering from such skin conditions as acne, eczema, psoriasis and cellulite. The sweating caused by deep heat helps eliminate dead skin cells, and improves skin tone and elasticity. Weight loss is facilitated through use of an infrared sauna – probably due to the increase in growth hormone that it produces. It has been calculated that one can burn 600 calories in 30 minutes in an infrared sauna. Health benefits can certainly be obtained in a

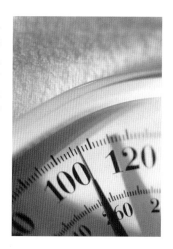

conventional sauna or steam bath as well, but the infrared sauna has a greater range of therapeutic efficiency, especially for detoxification. The infrared sauna actually has an energizing effect on users, making them feel good as toxins are eliminated.

Conventional saunas and steam baths are generally found in gymnasiums and health spas. Infrared saunas are more apt to be found in clinics run by holistic practitioners. People with health problems should consult a natural health care practitioner before using either type of sauna.

If you don't have access to a sauna or steam bath, you may want to do your own detoxification bath at home. This is prepared by filling a clean tub with hot filtered water (a shower filter or whole house filter is recommended) – as hot as you can comfortably tolerate. There are a number of therapeutic substances that can be used in the bath water. One is epsom salts, which contain magnesium to relax muscles and sulfur to aid in detoxification and help increase blood supply to the skin. A 1/4 cup of salts is a good start with a gradual increase to as much as two to four pounds per bath. Another option is ginger root. Ginger helps the body to sweat, so toxins are drawn to the skin's surface. To prepare the ginger bath, place half-inch slices of fresh ginger in boiling water; turn off the heat, and steep for 30 minutes. Remove the ginger, and pour the water into the tub.[2]

7

Dr. Hal Huggins suggests the following procedure for a detox bath:

- Bring the bath water to a temperature of 104 degrees Fahrenheit.
- Soak a bath sheet (3' x 6' towel) in the bath water.
- Get in the tub, and pull the bath sheet over you like you would a bed sheet.
- Keep the towel warm by periodically soaking it in the water.
- Leave the tub when you start to feel woozy.
- Stay in no longer than 20 minutes.
- Rinse off with fresh water.
- Repeat the procedure 2–3 times per week.

Dr. Huggins states that a soak of only two to three minutes will actually produce results, while benefits are maximized at 20 minutes. Often metals leave the body and appear after the bath in the form of a powder that adheres to the tub walls. Dr. Huggins suggests that adding a cup of baking soda to the bath water will enhance the effect of the soak. After the third bath, decrease baking soda to 1/2 cup, but also add 1/2 cup of Epsom salts. After another three baths, add 1 full cup of each.[3]

Other detox bath additives may include:

- Apple cider vinegar
- Hydrogen peroxide
- Clay
- Oatstraw (good for skin conditions)

In addition to saunas and detox baths, toxins may be eliminated from the skin by brushing it with a special natural bristle skin brush. This can be purchased in a health food store. Brush the skin before showering or bathing, stroking toward the heart, gently but vigorously. This will help stimulate lymph flow, as well as remove dead skin cells.

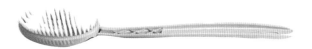

Colon Hydrotherapy

It is in the colon that the digestive process is completed; certain vitamins are synthesized, and water-soluble nutrients are absorbed. This important organ not only eliminates solid waste but also helps protect the body from infection and disease (a function of the beneficial flora). Dysbiosis can develop here, adversely affecting both elimination and overall health.

The importance of a high fiber diet, including plenty of fruits (unless Candida is an issue), vegetables and whole grains, has been explored, as has the advisability of using a balanced (soluble/insoluble) fiber supplement, especially when actively involved in a cleansing program. There is yet another way that the colon can be helped in its elimination process, and that is mechanically through the application of **colon hydrotherapy**.

Hydrotherapy is water therapy. Colon hydrotherapy then is the therapeutic application of water in the colon. The most familiar form of colon hydrotherapy is the enema. This mundane therapy has a most interesting history. Enema use dates to ancient Egypt; in fact, it is mentioned in the writings of several cultures in antiquity, including the Sumerians, Chinese, Hindus, Greeks and Romans.

Initially, enemas were a tool of the medical community, administered under the supervision of physicians. The practice of taking enemas (then called '**clysters**') became quite popular in the 17th century. The fluid carried in the clyster was often embellished with color and fragrance, and it was not uncommon for people to have as many as three to four daily rectal infusions. Monarchs were particularly privileged in this regard: History records that Louis XIII received more than 200 enemas in one year! As time passed, 'enema mania' faded, improvements were made in the process, and, by the early 19th century, colon hydrotherapy became once again the province of the medical community.

It was J.H. Kellogg, MD, of Battle Creek, Michigan (and Corn Flakes fame), who popularized colon hydrotherapy in the U.S. He reported in 1917 in the *Journal of the American Medical Association* that he was able to successfully treat all but 20 of 40,000 gastrointestinal patients using only diet, exercise and enemas – no surgery.

Dr. Kellogg's published success with enemas led to the development of advanced colon cleansing equipment to perform the colon-cleansing procedures known as **colonics** or **colonic irrigations**. A colonic is basically an extended and more complete form of an enema. Both the enema and the colonic involve the infusion of water into the rectum. However, the enema, is a one-time infusion; the patient takes in as much as a quart of water, holds it for a time, and then evacuates directly into

> *Since 1976, when colon hydrotherapy equipment has been registered with the FDA, there have been over 5 million colonics administered. Additionally, in this time, there has not been one verified or validated case, or any litigation alleging injury or death as a result of the use of the colon hydrotherapy equipment from the manufacturers of colon hydrotherapy equipment that are registered with the FDA.*
>
> - In a letter from I-ACT to the California Attorney General

the toilet. In contrast, colonic treatment (now known as colon hydrotherapy) involves repeated infusions of filtered, warm water into the colon by a certified colon therapist, while the gowned patient lies comfortably on a treatment table.

While water is sent through the sigmoid (only a small portion of the lower colon) with an enema, the water from a colonic travels throughout all sections of the large intestine. The colon therapist is trained to use massage techniques to relax abdominal muscles and ensure that all areas of the colon are adequately flushed. While the colon is filled and emptied a few times during one session (during a period of approximately 45 minutes), there is no need for the client to leave the table to expel the water: The passage of the water in and out of the colon is controlled by the therapist who operates the instrument. The client lies still as the water is expelled from the body. It travels through a clear viewing tube, which allows one to see what is being eliminated from the body – fecal matter, gas, mucus etc. There is no odor or health risk involved in the colonic procedure when performed properly by a trained practitioner. The therapeutic benefits of colon hydrotherapy are numerous and include:

- Improved muscle tone
- Reduced stagnation
- Reduced toxic waste absorption
- Thorough colon cleansing and balancing

7

Rheumatologist Arthur E. Brawer, MD, lists the following conditions among those he has found to respond well to colon hydrotherapy[4]:

- Allergies
- Arthritis
- Asthma
- Acne
- ADD
- Body odor
- Memory lapses
- Hypertension
- Chronic fatigue
- Brittle hair
- Brittle nails
- Spastic colon
- Cold hands and feet
- Colitis
- Headaches
- Multiple sclerosis
- Constipation
- Fibromyalgia
- Irritable bowel
- Mouth sores
- Nausea
- Peripheral neuropathies
- Peptic ulcer
- Potbelly
- Poor posture
- Seizures
- Muscle pain
- Joint aches
- Chest pain
- Skin rashes
- Toxic environmental exposure
- Toxic occupational exposure
- Pigmentation

Because of its many health benefits, colon hydrotherapy flourished in the U.S. until the mid-1960s, at which time it began a slow decline. By about 1972, most colonic equipment had been removed from hospitals and nursing homes, displaced by the use of drugs (prescriptive laxatives) and surgery (colostomy). Today, 100,000 such operations are performed annually (many of them unsuccessfully), while 70 million Americans who suffer from bowel problems are spending more than $400,000,000 every year on laxatives, according to the International Association for Colon Hydrotherapy.

> **Now, at the turn of the millennium, progressive physicians are turning once again to the use of colon hydrotherapy as an adjunct to their treatment protocols.**

A number of physicians using colon hydrotherapy (including gastroenterologists) were interviewed by Dr. Morton Walker for the August/September 2000 edition of *Townsend Letter for Doctors and Patients*. Their comments appear in his article entitled "Value of Colon Hydrotherapy Verified by Medical Professionals Prescribing It." The physicians interviewed by Dr. Walker presented case histories and spoke of the ability of colon hydrotherapy (used alone or in conjunction with other natural treatment modalities) to ease or resolve symptoms in people suffering from benign prostatic hyperplasia, cancer, silicone toxicity, diverticulosis, diverticulitis, yeast problems, drug and alcohol addiction and other disorders. Dr. James P. Carter, M.D., flatly stated that "it [colon hydrotherapy] takes away any desire to use drugs or imbibe in alcoholic beverages...should be part of nearly any addict's therapeutic regimen."[5] W. John Diamond, MD made the point that colon hydrotherapy stimulates the liver, thus helping to rid the body of debris that's sticking to the mucosa in the bowel wall.

Many patients have been able to overcome chronic constipation problems through colon hydrotherapy. Unlike chemical laxatives, which encourage dependency, colon hydrotherapy actually helps to tone the bowel, so that it resumes normal function. Hydrotherapy sessions can be used to 're-educate' the bowel to function normally. The International Association for Colon Hydrotherapy (I-ACT), headquartered in San Antonio, TX, is the worldwide certifying body for colon hydrotherapists. The organization works in conjunction with local municipalities to regulate the practice by establishing training standards and guidelines. I-ACT literature describes colon hydrotherapy as follows:

...a safe, effective method of removing waste from the large intestine, without the use of drugs. By introducing pure, filtered and temperature-regulated water into the colon, human waste is softened and loosened, resulting in evacuation through natural peristalsis.

> **To find an I-ACT certified colon hydrothera-pist who is using FDA registered equipment, disposable rectal nozzles (speculums) and fil-tered water, contact I-ACT at 210-366-2888 (www.i-act.org).**

Some people have concerns about colon hydrotherapy due to opinions expressed in articles (from some medical doctors and others) about the possibility of passing on disease and/or punctur-ing the colon. Such concerns are unfounded. A qualified therapist uses disposable tubes and speculums. The colonic instrument is FDA registered, so there are checks and balances to ensure its safety. As far as puncturing the colon, there is no basis for this concern. Colon hydrotherapy has been certified in the state of Florida since 1952 with no problems whatsoever. If properly per-formed, colon therapy is a safe healing modality. Some people have made statements questioning the safety of colon hydrotherapy. Such statements are usually opinions expressed by people who do not have all of the information; or their docu-mented 'evidence' should be thoroughly studied.

There are two types of FDA registered colon therapy instruments in the U.S. marketplace. These are referred to as 'open' and 'closed' systems. Switching from one system to another can cause some confusion for the layman.

The **closed system** is always operated by a thera-pist. The client is gowned and draped, and a speculum (rectal tube) is inserted in his rectum. He then turns over on his back. The therapist will fill the colon with water and empty it a number of times. The temperature of the water and the filling and emptying of the colon is always controlled by the therapist. The reason it is called a 'closed' system is that the water and waste material are always enclosed in tubing and instru-mentation. The waste material is disposed of through a closed drain system. The Resource Directory lists manufacturers of closed systems.

In the **open system**, the client is appropriately draped. Once the rectal tube is inserted, the ther-apist turns on the water. In some cases, the client may request privacy and conduct the colon thera-py session himself. The open system is best described as having a single tube bringing water into the colon. The waste material flows around the tube into the base of the instrument and is expelled into the sewer. An odor exhaust system ensures the room remains odor free. The Resource Directory lists manufacturers of open systems.

A final step to improve eliminations is to simulate the natural squatting posture while sitting on the toilet. This can be done by elevating the feet, rest-ing them on a special platform called a Life Step™ (see product insert).

Fasting/Juice Diets
Fasting is the abstinence from food for a period of time for therapeutic or religious purposes. This

supports the body by resting the digestive system and releasing energy for the body to use elsewhere. A short-term fast can last for one to three days. Longer than this would be considered long-term fasting. A water fast is not recommended unless supervised by a doctor. Toxins stored in the body begin to be released and could cause severe detox reactions. Also, people with blood sugar problems could be adversely affected. Most people can adequately and safely maintain a detoxification program based on juicing fresh fruits and vegetables. These supply the nutrients needed to support the body, and they require very little digestion. A juice diet is preferable to a water fast in today's toxic world.

Although it is unreasonable to eat 10 to 20 pounds of vegetables, it is easy to consume the juice from 10 to 20 pounds of vegetables during the course of a day. Even if the average person *were* able to eat that many vegetables, 90% or more of the nutrients would be eliminated in the vegetable fiber as it passes through the body. Juicing provides the full value – 100% – of the nutrients since the juice, containing all the nutrients, is normally separated from the vegetable fiber by the juicer. Freshly prepared juices are quickly and easily digested and absorbed in approximately 1/2 hour.

There are many good juicers on the market today, priced from about $40 to more than $1,000. The more expensive ones are more efficient; however, even the least expensive juicer on the market will work nicely for the person new to juicing.

There are also many fine books about juicing available in most local health food stores. We recommend *Juicing for Life* by Cherie Calbom and Maureen Keane. Both of these authors have master's degrees in nutrition and provide the reader not only with tasty, easy to prepare juice recipes, but also a great deal of useful information on which juices and nutrients are most useful in treating some 50 disorders, including a number of GI problems. They recommend consuming two to four glasses of freshly prepared juice daily. 'Fresh' is the key word here. As previously mentioned, juices begin to lose their nutritional value within a short time of extraction and therefore should be consumed immediately. They do not store well. The reason that juices from the supermarket stay 'fresh' is that they have been pasteurized to increase their shelf life. Usually chemical additives are used as well. There is no comparison between canned or bottled juices and freshly prepared juices. The former are nutrient-depleted and toxic to some degree because of the chemical residues they leave in the body; freshly prepared juices are rich in vitamins, minerals, enzymes and all the companion nutrients.

Step one in juicing is to buy the produce. Select organic produce, and wash it in hydrogen peroxide or a commercial veggie wash. If organic produce is unavailable, you may want to peel vegetables before running them through your juicer. The skins of most fruits and vegetables, including lemons and limes, may be left on. The skins of oranges, grapefruit, kiwis and papayas should be discarded, however. Remove pits from peaches, plums, etc., but fruits with seeds may be run through a juicer. An exception is apple seeds; these contain some cyanide so should be removed. Carrot and rhubarb greens must also be removed before juicing, as these contain toxic substances.

Any high water-content fruit or vegetable may be used in a juicer. This would include all fruit except bananas and avocados.

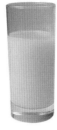

Drink four glasses (4–12 ounces each) of *fresh* juice throughout the day while on a juice diet. Also, you'll want to drink at least four 8-ounce glasses of water throughout the day.

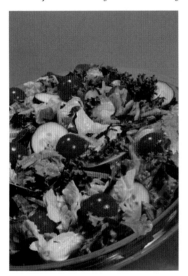

How you end a juice diet is just as important as sticking to the diet. It is imperative to ease into normal eating. The first meal after a juice diet is concluded may consist of a fruit or vegetable salad with lemon juice dressing, accompanied by juice and herbal tea. The second meal could consist of the salad plus a fresh vegetable soup, plus juice. The same items could be repeated for dinner – or a steamed vegetable may be substituted for the soup. On the second day, breakfast would be the same: juice, salad and herbal tea. Lunch might consist of juice, salad, soup and brown rice. By dinner of the second day, a potato and baked or broiled fish may be added. Ending a juice diet too quickly, with the wrong foods, can put an extra load on the body and cancel the benefits gained. This is very important to keep in mind.

Prolonged juice diets may be used therapeutically under supervision to treat serious disorders. The late Max Gerson, MD, was noted for his success with treating cancer patients, using juice therapy (13 glasses per day!) as a focal point of treatment.

A juice diet is not required to detoxify the body, and for some people, may not be feasible. Others may want to start their cleansing program with a couple of days of fresh juice; the weekend would be the best time so there is time for adequate rest. Apart from juice diets, adding fresh juice to a daily diet will support a cleansing program. The simpler the better!

> While fresh vegetable juices are highly nourishing, and a periodic juice diet can be very beneficial in ridding the body of toxins, don't substitute juice for vegetables after the diet is completed. You may certainly add juice to your diet (and are encouraged to do so), but don't exclude the veggies: The body needs the fiber provided by whole foods.

Nutrient Supplementation

Those on a detoxification program can benefit from extra vitamins and minerals, particularly the antioxidants (vitamins A, C, E and the minerals selenium and zinc), as well as B vitamins. A multi-vitamin and mineral may be used to support the body as it is detoxifying toxic chemicals. Make super foods, such as green drinks, a regular part of your diet. Green food drinks provide an excellent supply of nutrients during and after a detox program. They can help to boost energy during the day. The Resource Directory includes sources for some excellent green food supplements.

7

Exercise/Deep Breathing

Exercise is an important element in a health-building regimen. It is also very important in the detoxification process. When we breathe in and

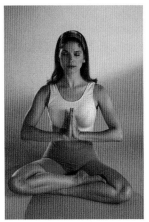

out, the flow of lymph through the body is stimulated. It has long been known that exercise stimulates this movement of lymphatic fluid, but the role of breathing wasn't entirely recognized until technology provided the means to photograph the lymph flow process. This direct observation shows that deep breathing causes the lymph to shoot through the capillaries like a geyser. The key word here is 'deep.' *Deep* breathing is the kind that best stimulates lymph flow. Breathing deeply helps eliminate poisons from the cells, and also enhances immunity, since the lymphatic system is actually part of the immune system. Deep breathing enhances immunity by eliminating toxins. While the heart is the pump for the vascular system, the lymphatic system has no real pump: It depends upon movement (exercise) and breath for stimulation. Properly used, the lungs act as sort of a suction pump for the lymphatic system.

Combining deep breathing with exercise – even gentle exercise like jumping on a rebounder (mini-trampoline) – will do much to improve lymph flow and thus the body's detoxification ability and general state of health. Yoga is another tool to stimulate lymph flow, one that focuses upon stretching and controlled breathing. It's empowering to know that something as simple and (free) as breathing, can be used as a powerful tool to build health. ⚜

Notes

[1] Hal Huggins, DDS, MS, *Detoxification*, Peak Energy Performance, p. 19.

[2] Cheryl Townsley, *Cleaning Made Simple*, LFH Publishing, 1997, p. 47-48.

[3] Ibid., p. 23.

[4] Morton Walker, "Value of Colon Hydrotherapy Verified by Medical Professionals Prescribing it," *Townsend Letter for Doctors and Patients*, August/September, 2000 (#205/ 206), p. 4.

[5] Ibid., p. 6.

Chapter Summary - Recommended Actions

When you start a detox (cleansing) program, especially as a first-time cleanser, it is important to keep it simple. A realistic commitment is required to stay excited about creating long-term optimal health. Some detox options may not be available to you, or you may not be able to fit them into your schedule. The whole-body herbal cleansing program is not a one-time affair. It is best incorporated into a prevention program at least twice a year. It is the first step toward complete detoxification. Again, for people who have many health problems, it may be necessary to seek the services of a natural health care practitioner or physician who can design a custom program. Regardless of whether you choose this option or elect to use a pre-formulated cleanse, this is your first step in the detoxification process, the cornerstone of good health. Whichever option is chosen, clean the digestive system, and support the organs of elimination before moving on to more advanced cleanses, like those that address Candida, parasites, heavy metals or liver detoxification. A simplified 30-day whole-body cleanse would look like this:

1. Maintain a 'clean,' healthy diet, one which excludes refined starches and includes the following:

   • Plenty of fresh organic fruits and vegetables

- Organic meat, used as a condiment (2 1/2-ounce per meal for women, 3 1/2–4-ounce per meal for men).
- Ezekiel bread (sprouted whole grain)
- Herbal teas
- Purified water (with minerals added back) – 7 to 10 glasses daily
- Fresh juices (optional)
- Cold-pressed (unrefined) olive oil
- Real butter

2. Take an herbal detox formula (which contains herbs discussed in this chapter) morning and night for 30 days. To help support the body in the cleansing process during this time, also add:

    a. Essential oils after breakfast and dinner (one to two capsules)
    b. A balanced flax fiber supplement before bed
    c. Vitamins, minerals after meals
    d. Super foods such as green drinks
    e. Plant enzymes (containing HCl, if necessary) with meals.

3. Skin brush.

4. Take a hot therapeutic bath, steam bath or sauna three times a week.

5. Try colon hydrotherapy at least three times or more during the 30–day detox.

6. Exercise for 30 minutes: walking, yoga or rebounder.

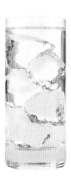
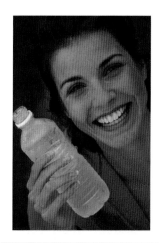

FACT: 75% of Americans are chronically dehydrated. (Likely applies to half the world population)

FACT: In 37% of Americans, the thirst mechanism is so weak that it is often mistaken for hunger.

FACT: Even *mild* dehydration will slow down one's metabolism as much as 3%.

FACT: One glass of water stopped midnight hunger pains for almost 100% of the dieters in a University of Washington study.

FACT: Lack of water is the #1 trigger of daytime fatigue.

FACT: Preliminary research indicates that 8–10 glasses of water a day could significantly ease back and joint pain for as much as 80% of sufferers.

FACT: A mere 2% drop in body water can trigger fuzzy short-term memory, trouble with basic math and difficulty focusing on the computer screen or on a printed page.

7

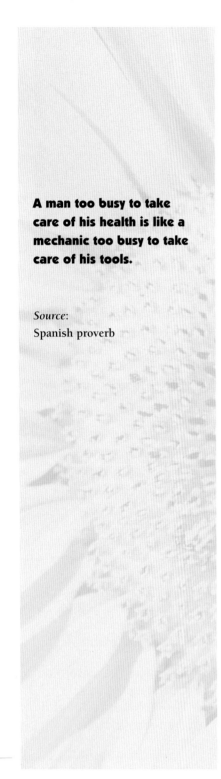

CHAPTER 8

BALANCING gut flora
/Repairing the Intestinal Mucosa

BALANCING GUT FLORA

The intestinal tract contains more than 500 species of bacteria. It is critical to good health and the immune system that the right ratio of good bacteria to bad bacteria (80%:20%) be maintained in the intestines. If the bad, or in some cases even benign microorganisms (yeast) are prevalent, a condition called dysbiosis can occur. There are many causes of dysbiosis. It is usually self-induced, meaning it results from high levels of stress, chemical exposure, poor diet, overuse of antibiotics, birth control pills and/or drugs of all kinds. The over-prescribing of antibiotics is probably the single most responsible factor for imbalance in the digestive tract. There are ways to balance the gut flora with advanced cleansing methods. In order to establish bacterial balance, one will need to:

• Eliminate Candida, if present.
• Eliminate parasites, if present.
• Reestablish good bacteria.

In order to determine if Candida is a problem for you, we have included in the appendix a self-scoring questionnaire. You may also want to use one of the labs listed in the Resource Directory. They perform a specialized stool analysis to determine if you have Candida or parasites. You will need to consult a holistic physician or health care practitioner to have the test performed. I have found the questionnaire to be very effective in determining if one has Candida. In dealing with either problem, the following protocol is important and must be followed:

1. Eliminate the use of antibiotics, steroids, immunosuppressive drugs and oral contraceptives (only after consulting a health care provider).
2. Starve the yeast (with diet).
3. Exterminate the yeast (with natural anti-fungals).

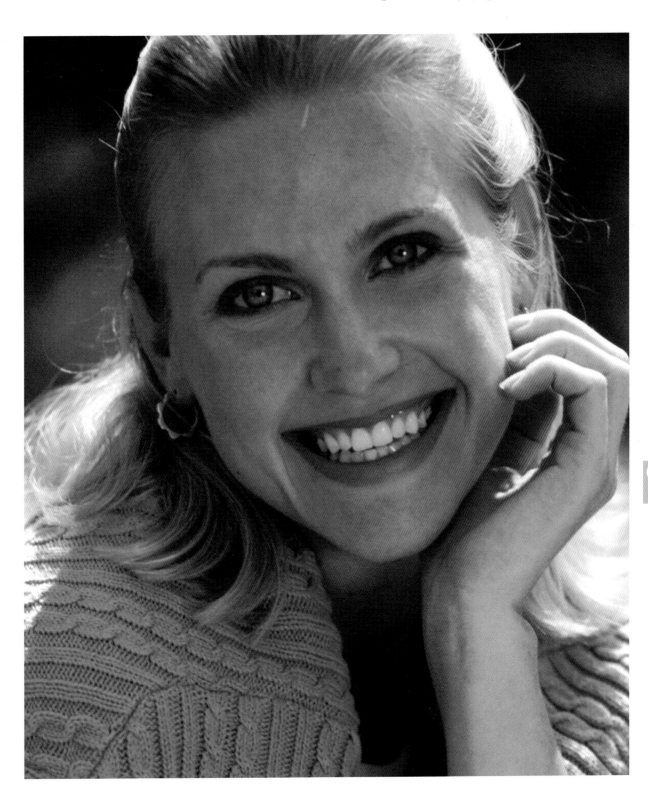

8

4. Kill parasites.

5. Replace the good bacteria.

6. Support the body, especially the immune
system, with supplemental nutrients.

The Diet

The diet outlined here is an eating plan, not a typical diet with specific foods, quantities or eating
schedules. It provides guidelines for creating
healthy, appealing meals. For better results from
this diet, avoid certain medications such as birth
control pills (the result of eliminating birth control
pills can be pregnancy), cortisone-type drugs and
antibiotics, as these medications will promote dysbiosis in the gut, making it difficult to normalize
the Candida population. If these medications are
necessary, then postpone the diet (indeed, the
whole Candida program) until the medications are
stopped. Avoid any known food allergens, even if
they are listed as permissible foods in the diet.

This diet features an abundance of fresh
organic vegetables and lean organic low- and
medium-stress meats (fish and poultry primarily).
The high-stress proteins (peanuts, non-fermented
soy, pork lamb, veal beef, commercial cow milk)
should be temporarily avoided while cleansing,
and eaten in moderation afterwards. These are the
proteins that take the most energy to digest.

Attention

If you have followed anti-Candida programs
in the past without success, consult your
natural health care practitioner/dentist to rule
out oral focal infection and/or heavy metal
toxicity, with the aid of appropriate lab tests
(see Resource Directory) as discussed in
chapter 4.

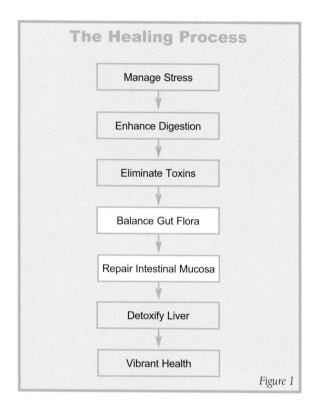

Figure 1

Among the vegetables, the diet emphasizes those
low in starch (the green leafies, primarily), though
the starchy vegetables (lima beans, peas, potatoes,
etc.) may be eaten in small amounts.

The goal of this diet is to avoid anything that will
either feed the yeast or otherwise contribute to
its growth. Molds, mildew, fungi – these are all
relatives of Candida and are to be avoided,
as exposure to them places an extra burden on
the immune system. One common source of mold
is that which grows on leftovers placed in the
refrigerator. Foods so stored deteriorate rapidly
(within 24 hours), supporting the growth of
molds and bacteria. Leftovers should be frozen
– OR vacuum sealed before refrigerating to retard
oxidation (spoiling). Vacuum packaged food
items will keep fresh at least three to five times
longer than conventionally packaged food items
when placed in the refrigerator or freezer.

(Tilia, Inc., at 1-877-804-5383, www.foodsaver.com, has information on home vacuum packaging systems.)

Donna Gates' excellent book, *The Body Ecology Diet,* provides more detail on Candida and has some great recipes. Another fine book on Candida, which gives carbohydrate (and calorie) content of foods and some very good recipes (complete with pre-calculated carbohydrate totals) and information, is Pat Connolly's *The Candida Albicans Yeast-Free Cookbook*. This book also contains a 'cheats and treats' section. The author is curator of the Price-Pottenger Nutrition Foundation, a non-profit educational organization dedicated to making the works of nutrition experts like the late Weston A. Price, DDS, and the late Francis M. Pottenger, Jr., MD, and others available to the public. PPNF information is available at 1-800-366-3748 (www.price pottenger.org).

While limiting carbohydrates is important to the success of the diet, especially in the first week, it is also important not to eliminate them *totally* from the diet. An intake of less than 60 grams of carbohydrates a day is not recommended because of the macronutrient imbalance that could result.

The following dietary modifications for exterminating Candida are recommended:

1. **Eliminate sugars and artificial sweeteners**, as well as foods containing them. This includes sucrose (or table sugar), honey, fructose, molasses, maple syrup and other concentrated sweeteners. A moderate amount of the herbs stevia or lo han may be used as a sweetener when needed.

2. **Limit grains**. All grains should be totally eliminated during the first week or two of the diet. Those that do not contain gluten (corn, millet, teff, quinoa) may be added later. Only whole grains are recommended, used sparingly – no more than four servings daily (1/2–1 cup = a serving).

3. **Avoid fruits and fruit juices**, except for Granny Smith apples. Lemon juice may be used in herb tea or water. If fruit is a 'must have' for some reason, then sub-acids, like a few strawberries or blueberries, can be included.

4. **Avoid all canned and frozen juices**. Stick with freshly prepared vegetable juices (see next section).

5. **Avoid yeast-containing foods**. This includes most types of bread (and rolls and crackers). A variety of yeast-free breads is generally available at natural food stores. Use these in moderation. Beer, wine and other alcoholic beverages also contain yeast and should therefore be avoided, as should sauerkraut, commercial salad dressings, all types of vinegars, soy sauce, Worcestershire sauce, horseradish, pickles, relish, green olives, commercial soups, potato chips and dry roasted nuts. Try olive oil (or flax oil) and lemon juice as a salad dressing.

8

6. **Avoid mushrooms and all types of cheeses**. These either contain or actually *are* molds or yeasts.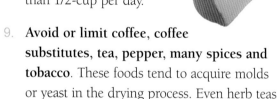

7. **Avoid peanuts and peanut butter**. These have a high content of afla-toxins, a carcinogenic mold. Almond butter, cashew butter, tahini (sesame seed butter) or other nut or seed butters may be substituted. These should be refrigerated to avoid rancidity. Raw nuts and seeds make good snacks when soaked overnight in water to make them more digestible.

8. **Avoid commercial dairy products**. The exceptions are butter and plain (*not* low-fat or no-fat) yogurt, in small amounts – no more than 1/2-cup per day.

9. **Avoid or limit coffee, coffee substitutes, tea, pepper, many spices and tobacco**. These foods tend to acquire molds or yeast in the drying process. Even herb teas may become moldy, so their use should be limited, especially for sensitive individuals. Teas with anti-fungal properties include pau d'arco, chamomile, bergamot, hyssop, alfalfa, angelica root and lemon grass.[1] Pau d' arco, in particular, has been shown to be effective in killing Candida.

10. **Avoid meat, fish and poultry that is pick-led, smoked or dried**. This includes smoked salmon, oysters, sardines, hot dogs, salami, corned beef, ham, bacon and pastrami.[2]

While many fermented foods, such as sauerkraut and tempeh (a fermented soy bean product), are restricted, there are a few that are permitted – plain yogurt (in small amounts), raw unfiltered cider vinegar and cultured vegetables (described later in this chapter).

We suggest you cook with olive oil and use it as a salad dressing, as it has a high content of oleic acid, which has been found to prevent the conversion of Candida to its fungal form. Unrefined extra virgin olive oil is the best choice.

We realize this is a long list of foods to avoid, but many others are *permissible* including:

- Low starch vegetables
- Legumes (soaked and cooked at low temperatures)
- Good quality lean meats (organic)
- Nuts and seeds (soaked overnight in distilled or purified water)
- Green vegetable juices (Fruit has too much sugar; carrots should not be used alone.)
- Granny Smith apples
- Lo han or stevia (used in moderation) as a sweetener
- Gluten/yeast-free breads
- Raw almond butter
- Pasta (quinoa or rice)
- Plain yogurt or keifer, unsweetened (in moderation)
- Hot air popcorn (in moderation)
- Eggs (if not sensitive)

There really are a number of tasty dishes that can be prepared using these foods – just pick up a Candida cookbook and see. Emphasize soups and salads. There is no limit to how much of these you may eat.

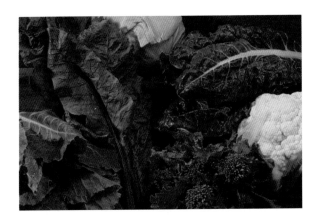

You'll do well to include plenty of green vegetables and their juices, for these have a high content of chlorophyll. Chlorophyll, in concentrated amounts, is "known to inhibit bacteria and relieve many of the discomforts of candidiasis – itching, burning, gas, bloating."[3] You'll also want to use plenty of garlic in your diet, as this food is well known as a natural antibiotic. It is also anti-fungal due to its **allicin** content. If you use a garlic supplement, make sure it contains this important ingredient. Many deodorized garlics do not. Other anti-Candida agents that may be used liberally include ginger, cinnamon, thyme and rosemary.

Children may follow the same basic diet, but without the strict prohibition of starches. Limited amounts of whole grains and fruits may be consumed. Refined sugars and fruit juices, however, should be absolutely avoided. It would also be well for children to stay away from wheat and other common allergens, at least initially.

There is no set rule about duration of this diet. It should be followed for at least three months. The severity of the infestation and how much 'cheating' is done during the diet will also dictate how long an individual stays on the diet. Generally speaking, when symptoms have subsided, foods may be slowly added back, starting with fruits, then grains (wheat last) and dairy products. Add

---

Please Note

It is suggested that people with Candida, as well as anyone who has moved on the Health Continuum towards 'toxic overload,' follow this diet for a period of time. Many who have Candida may eventually develop food sensitivities, fibromyalgia and other chronic problems.

foods back one at a time. If old symptoms return or gas and bloating occur, then resume the diet, for this is a sign that the yeast has been re-activated. The use of potent anti-fungal herbs could well lessen the duration of the diet, possibly to as little as one month. However, it is important to ease off the diet regimen and settle into a good maintenance dietary plan, following the guidelines presented in chapter 10. Returning to a junk food diet will defeat the purpose of the cleanse.

During the cleanse, you may experience discomfort as the yeast dies off. Symptoms may include headaches, food cravings, nausea, body aches, irritability, etc. Using powdered vitamin C (the buffered variety, 1/8–1/2 teaspoon in water between meals) or L-glutamine may help with these reactions.

While on a Candida cleanse, you'll want to prepare your own food as much as possible. This requires planning and more planning. This diet will only succeed if you are prepared to reduce hunger with appropriate foods and snacks. Have a back-up plan prepared and a restaurant selected that can prepare food 'to go' in case of emergency.

8

When you eat out, order plain foods. Avoid those with sauces, as they may contain sugar and vinegar. You'll also want to avoid charcoal-grilled foods and rolled deli meats. The best choices are fresh vegetables (a la carte), if available, or a vegetable relish plate. For a salad dressing, ask for olive oil and a slice of lemon. Sparkling water with a wedge of lemon is the beverage of choice. No desserts, of course.

If fibromyalgia, arthritis or inflammation has developed, then 'nightshades' may have to be removed from the diet. The nightshade group includes:

- Tomatoes
- Peppers of all kinds (red, green, yellow, chili, paprika, cayenne, hot/sweet)
- Potatoes
- Pimentos
- Eggplant
- Tobacco

According to Gloria Gilbére, in the book *Invisible Illnesses*, removing nightshades from the diet can really help with inflammation.

Juicing
Below are a few of the recipes for candidiasis from an excellent and informative book on juicing by Calbom and Keane[4]:

Ginger Hopper
1/4" slice ginger root
4–5 carrots, greens removed
1/2 apple, seeded [Granny Smith variety]

Push ginger thru hopper with carrots & apple.

Potassium Broth
Handful parsley
Handful spinach
5 carrots, greens removed
3 stalks celery

Bunch up parsley & spinach leaves, and push through hopper with carrots and celery.

Cherie's Cleansing Cocktail
1/4" slice ginger root
1 beet
1/2 apple, seeded [Granny Smith variety]
4 carrots, greens removed

Push ginger, beet & apple thru hopper with carrots.

High-Calcium Drink
3 kale leaves
Small handful parsley
4–5 carrots, greens removed

Bunch up kale & parsley, & push thru hopper with carrots.

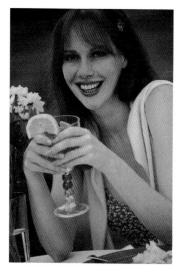

Calbom and Keene list vitamin B6, selenium, iron and zinc as key nutrients for fighting Candida and tell us which vegetables contain high amounts of each:[5]

Vitamin B6:	kale, spinach, turnip greens
Selenium:	red Swiss chard, turnip, garlic, radish
Iron:	parsley, beet greens, dandelion greens, broccoli
Zinc:	ginger root, parsley, garlic, carrot

Natural Anti-fungal Cleansing Programs
A formulation with a very broad spectrum of anti-fungal agents is highly recommended. Such a formula will target many different types of yeast

organisms. The program should be followed for at least 15 to 30 days while adhering to the diet previously described. Those who have previously been treated for Candida may have used a single anti-fungal agent (such as caprylic acid). Some yeast organisms can become resistant to that agent, much like bacteria resist antibiotics. A great choice for those who have been exposed

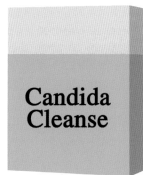

to other anti-fungal agents is a formula with a wide variety of ingredients that will compensate for, or override, any resistance that may have developed to a single anti-fungal agent. Such a formula would contain a wide spectrum of compounds known to be effective in eradicating yeast as well as compounds that kill amoebae.

A 2-part detox kit matching the above description is designed with simplicity in mind: Capsules and a liquid tincture in the morning and before bed can fit into anyone's schedule.

Ideally, the following anti-fungal agents would be used:

- **Uva ursi** – shown in Germany to be effective in eliminating Candida
- **Calcium undecylenate** – (comes from the castor bean) has been shown to be six times more effective than caprylic acid in killing yeast.
- **Neem leaf** – contains strong antibiotic alkaloids and tannins.
- **Olive leaf** – a traditional anti-fungal
- **Berberine sulphate** – a concentrated anti-fungal/anti-bacterial compound found in barberry
- **Oregon grape root** – contains berberine, a strong anti-fungal/antibacterial.

- **Oregano leaf** – contains the alkaloids carvacrol and thymol, both of which are strong anti-fungals.

An important component of any advanced cleansing program is fiber. As noted, flax fiber (organic) is the best choice. Such fiber, formulated with combinations of slippery elm and marshmallow, will soothe the irritated colon.

A digestive enzyme formula for supporting the proper digestion of food is also needed in an advanced cleansing program. With Candida and other conditions, most people have low HCl in the stomach, which is what causes the pH to be unbalanced. A formula with HCl, glutamine and N-acetyl-glucosamine supports the intestinal lining.

Eliminate Parasites

Parasite elimination is critical for balancing the gut flora. In some cases, parasites can be detected with stool analysis. This can be tricky due to the life cycle of parasites. Candida and parasites tend to appear together, so when a Candida program has not been successful, it might be appropriate to try a different approach, one that uses a natural product that concentrates on both parasites and Candida. Anti-parasitic herbs work by using three different mechanisms: One group paralyzes the microorganism directly, which allows the body to remove it through the regular channels of the digestive system. This type of action is specific to **nematode** (worm) type organisms. Another group directly destroys the organism so that it can be removed from the body through the GI tract. Others work by stimulating the body's own natural processes to eliminate the organism – i.e., stimulating the secretion of HCl. Anti-fungals work by directly eroding the cell wall of yeast/fungal organisms, which debilitates them or makes them more susceptible to destruction by the friendly bacteria in the GI tract.

A natural anti-parasitic product should contain key ingredients like:

- Black walnut (an extract made from the green rind of the hull) – This is more effective in a liquid tincture, as it needs to be processed quickly upon picking.
- Wormwood
- Cloves
- Garlic
- Undecylenic acid
- Grapefruit seed extract
- Pumpkin seed
- Pippli
- Quassia
- Rosemary and thyme

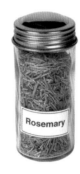

Such a formula usually comes in two parts – in a capsule and in a tincture. It should be taken three times daily for 15 days, then a 5-day break, followed by 15 days of use. This cycle can be repeated two to three times, depending upon severity. When undertaking a parasite cleanse, people often experience a wide range of symptoms.

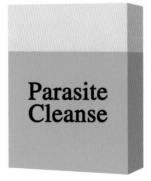

Some have increased energy, while others are fatigued. Some think more clearly, while others are less alert. Some may actually see parasites in the stool (even though most are microscopic); others do not. After 7 days, however, cleansing reactions usually start to subside.

While on the parasite cleanse, it would be best to follow the anti-Candida diet. Also, add flax fiber and a digestive enzyme with HCl, as with the Candida regimen. Some people do parasite cleanses as part of their prevention program or when they have traveled out of the country.

Replace Gut Flora

The next step in the process of balancing gut flora is to return the good bacteria to the digestive tract with a probiotic formula.

If, after stopping a Candida or parasite cleanse, the symptoms reoccur, then the good bacteria probably haven't been reestablished.

The term 'probiotics' comes from the Greek words, 'pro' and 'biotics,' meaning 'for life' or 'in favor of life.' Holistic practitioners often begin any discussion of probiotics with this very basic definition because of its simplicity and clarity. Probiotics are beneficial and even necessary to life. They are predominately bacterial; however, some fungi (like Saccharomyces boulardii) are also considered beneficial 'probiotic' microorganisms.

Resident vs. Transient Strains

Another important point about beneficial bacteria involves the relationship between resident and transient strains. Resident strains are those strains that are commonly found in the human digestive tract. Lactobacillus acidophilus and Bifidobacteria bifudum are common resident strains found virtually in all human intestinal systems. Lactobacillus casei, Lactobacillus bulgarius and Streptococcus thermophillus are common transient strains.

Transient strains are often consumed in foods like yogurt. These strains will not reestablish in the digestive tract; however, they do provide many benefits as they pass through.

Probiotics, Prebiotics and Synbiotics

Probiotics have been defined as living microorganisms that positively improve health and intestinal environment. A prebiotic is defined as "a non-digestible food ingredient that beneficially affects the host by selectively stimulating the growth and/or activity of one or a limited number of bacteria in the colon" (Gibson and Roberfroid, 1995). A prebiotic is further defined as a dietary ingredient that reaches the large intestine in an intact form and has a specific metabolism therein, one directed toward beneficial rather than harmful bacteria. A true prebiotic must:

1. be neither hydrolyzed nor absorbed by the upper part of the digestive tract
2. be a selective substrate for one or a limited number of beneficial bacteria
3. be able to alter the colonic flora in favor of a healthier composition
4. induce luminal or systemic effects that are beneficial to the host

Selecting The Probiotic

There are at least 100 companies distributing probiotic products today. It is interesting to note that there are far fewer companies (perhaps a dozen or so) that actually manufacture or culture the majority of the probiotics sold in the U.S. Companies (many of them quite large) contract with these manufactures to produce a specific proprietary formulation that serves the particular market they are attempting to support. Each probiotic formula will be different. The products will have different types

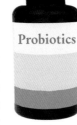

Probiotics

and numbers of cultures; they may or may not be packaged with a prebiotic, and they will have a broad range of prices. In order to make a selection, consider the following:

Species selection – The majority of studies have been conducted using species from either the Lactobacillus or Bifidobacteria family. These are the most prevalent beneficial genera. Since these genera have no known pathogenic species or strains, they are generally thought of as being the safest and most well-researched probiotics.

Transient vs. resident – Most probiotic products consist of multiple species from either the Lactobacilli or Bifidobacteria family. Some of the Lactobacilli species are transient bacteria (L. casei), and others are resident. While both

Resident Strains in Humans
Lactobacillus acidophilus
Lactobacillus salivarius
Bifidobacterium bifidum
Bifidobacterium infantis
Bifidobacterium longum
Streptococcus faecalis
Streptococcus faecium

Transient Strains
Lactobacillus brevis
Lactobacillus bulgaricus
Lactobacillus casei
Lactobacillus delbrueckii
Lactobacillus kefir
Lactobacillus plantarum
Lactobacillus yoghurti
Streptococcus lactis
Streptococcus thermophilus

Figure 2

8

Pro, Pre and Synbiotics

PROBIOTIC

Definition	A live microbial food supplement which beneficially affects the host animal by improving its intestinal microbial balance.
Examples	Lactobacilli, Bifidobacteria, Enterococci, Streptococci
Advantages	Strain may have proven health values. Useful when gut flora may be compromised
Possible Future Developments	New product developments based on synbiotics that may improve probiotic survival

PREBIOTIC

Definition	A non-digestible food ingredient that beneficially affects the host by selectively stimulating the growth and/or activity of one or a limited number of bacteria in the colon, and thus improves host health
Examples	Frutooligosaccharides (FOS), inulin, galactooligosaccharides
Advantages	Genus-level changes occur in gut flora. Product survival not problematic. Low dose required and can be incorporated into may different food delivery systems.
Possible Future Developments	Manufacture of novel mutiple-function prebiotics, that may: stimulate the 'beneficial' flora; exert anti-adhesive properties; attenuate pathogen virulence. Prebiotics derived from dietary fiber-type polysacchrides

SYNBIOTIC

Definition	A mixture of pro and pre-biotics which beneficially affects the host by improving the survival and implantation of live microbial dietary supplements in the gastrointestinal tract
Examples	Fruto-oligosaccharides (FOS), + bifidobacteria; lactitol + lactobacilli
Advantages	Dual effect of entities. Probiotic survival should be improved.
Possible Future Developments	Design of new synbiotics through molecular engineering (based on specific prebiotic enzymes)

Chart taken from *The Advanced Guide to Longevity Medicine* by Mitchell J. Ghen, p. 213

Figure 3

resident and transient species are beneficial, resident species may offer the advantage of reestablishment in the digestive tract. Resident species may also be more likely to work together and be less antagonistic to other resident strains already in the digestive tract. One strategy is to use a product that has multiple strains of resident Lactobacilli and Bifidobacteria species to rebuild and maintain the intestinal environment. Specific, well-tested transient strains (L. casei or L. bulgaricus) are then used individually to boost the maintenance dose.

Site Utilization – Species selection is also dependent on the area of the intestinal tract being targeted. Since it is often difficult to determine the specific intestinal area of need, a multi-species product that contains both Lactobacillus and Bifidobacteria may be the best choice because these species target both the small and large intestine.

Culture counts – Probiotics are usually measured in numbers of organisms per capsule, per tablet or per gram (in the case of powders). High-potency products typically contain two to four billion or more organisms in a capsule or tablet and four billion cultures per gram in the powder. All products should list an expiration date on the label, which would indicate how long the product will retain its stated potency.

Storage – Most of the common probiotic species, Lactobacillus acidophilus and Bifidobacterium bifidum, for example, do not survive for long periods at or above room temperatures. A few probiotics, like Streptococcus faecium, can survive at room temperatures. The problem is that manufacturers mix the species in the same formulation. Unrefrigerated organisms do not die immediately, but if probiotics that require refrigeration are stored on the shelf for weeks or months, the loss of potency can be significant. Even non-refrigerated species may retain potency longer in refrigeration. In general, refrigerated products should be refrigerated and mixed only with other refrigerated species. Non-refrigerated probiotics should be formulated only with other non-refrigerated species.

Prebiotics – There is significant research that supports the use of prebiotics in promoting enhanced levels of beneficial bacteria. Fructo-oligosaccharides (FOS) are added to many probiotic formulations. Prebiotics like FOS have been shown clinically to enhance the intestinal levels of beneficial probiotics. Selecting a formulation that contains multiple resident probiotics (Lactobacillus, Bifidobacterium) and prebiotics (FOS) is desirable.

Dosing The Probiotic.

There are two considerations in selecting the ideal dose of probiotics: The first is when to take the probiotic (with meals or between meals), and the second is how much to take.

Some practitioners suggest that taking probiotics with meals can aid in digestion. Others suggest that taking probiotics between meals, when stomach acid is lowest, is best. In general, probiotics taken once or twice daily with a large glass of water, between meals can help deliver the probiotic to the intestinal tract faster and in higher concentrations.

To maintain healthy levels of intestinal flora, two to four billion cultures daily are commonly recommended. For specific health issues, 10 to 15 billion cultures once or twice daily may be needed.

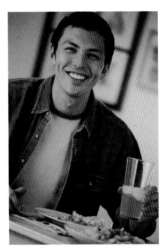

Research continues to support the holistic concept that achieving long term vibrant health is dependant on having balanced body systems that function together. The digestive system is one of the most important, and in some ways least understood, of these systems. A balanced intestinal environment is a critical component of any healthy digestive system. Practitioners today have a variety of new tools to use that can help them help their patients achieve improved digestive health. Probiotics, prebiotics, enzymes and amino compounds can be used to help maintain a healthy intestinal ecosystem and extended longevity.

Some Beneficial Microflora and their Characteristics

Lactobacillus acidophilus – is a natural bacteria that inhabits the small and large intestines of humans and animals, human mouth and vagina.

8

Facultative anaerobic lactobacilli (which grow in the presence or absence of air) produce lactic acid as a main product from carbohydrates. Their optimum growth temperature is 95°-100°F. The major beneficial functions of acido-bacteria are:

1. They enhance and allow digestion of milk sugar (lactose) by producing the enzyme lactase, and generally aid in the digestion of nutrients.
2. They are capable by some competitive means, by the creation of lactic acid and by other inhibitory substances, to suppress undesirable microorganisms in the intestines.
3. Some strains help to destroy hostile invading bacteria by producing natural antibiotic substances.
4. Some strains help to reduce the level of cholesterol, thus lessening the dangers of cardiovascular complications.
5. They help to lessen the proliferation of hostile yeast such as Candida albicans. When the intestinal microflora is disturbed (the lactobacilli adversely affected) under the influence of oral antibiotic therapy, or stress conditions, the use of supplemental acidophilus, in food or concentrated form, can help reverse such negative processes. The regular use of acidophilus bacteria, as a supplement or in food, is a protective measure against an imbalance of the intestinal microflora.

Bifidobacterium bifidum – is a natural inhabitant of the human intestines but also found in the human vagina. B. bifidum occurs in larger numbers in the large intestine than in the lower part of the intestine. They and other Bifidobacteria species are the predominant organisms in the large intestine of breast-fed infants, accounting for approximately 99% of the microflora. In adolescents and adults, Bifidobacteria are a major component of the large intestine's microflora. The level of Bifidobacteria declines with age and also in various conditions of ill-health. They produce acetic and lactic acid, with small amounts of formic acid from fermentable carbohydrates. They are anaerobic bacteria with an optimum growth temperature of 98°-105°F. The major beneficial functions are:

1. The prevention of the colonization of the intestines by invading pathogenic bacteria or yeast with which they compete for nutrients and attachment sites
2. The production of acetic and lactic acids that lower the pH of the intestines, thus making the region undesirable for other possibly harmful bacteria
3. Assist in nitrogen retention and weight gain in infants
4. The inhibition of bacteria that can alter nitrates in the intestines (derived from food or water) into potentially harmful nitrites
5. The production of B vitamins
6. Assist in the dietary management of liver conditions (When the intestinal microflora are disturbed – and consequently Bifidobacteria decline – under the influence of oral antibiotic therapy, therapeutic irradiation of the abdomen, reduced gastric acidity, impaired intestinal motility, stresses or some other conditions, Bifidobacteria supplements or Bifidobacteria found in food products, such as bifidus milk, can help to restore the intestinal microflora.)

Lactobacillus salivarius – bacteria are a natural resident of the human intestine and mouth. These are facultative anaerobic lacobacilli that produce lactic acid as a main product from carbohydrates. Their optimum growth temperature is 95°-104°F. As with other lactic acid bacteria, they encourage, because of their creation of lactic acid, a more acidic environment in which less desirable microorganisms are inhibited.

Bifidobacterium infantis – is a natural inhabitant of the intestines of human infants, but also occurs in small numbers in the human vagina. Together with other Bifidobacteria species, such as B. bifidum and B. longum, they are the predominant organisms in the large intestine of infants. They are anaerobic bacteria that produce acetic and lactic acids and small amounts of formic acid from carbohydrates. The major beneficial functions are similar to those of B. bifidum:

1. The prevention of the colonization of the intestines by invading pathogenic bacteria or yeast with which they compete for nutrients and attachments sites
2. The production of acetic and lactic acids that lower the pH of the intestines, thus making the region undesirable for other possibly harmful bacteria
3. Assist in nitrogen retention and weight gain in infants
4. The inhibition of bacteria, which can alter nitrates into potentially harmful nitrites
5. The production of B vitamins

When the intestinal microflora of infants is disturbed (and the levels of Bifidobacteria decline) under the influence of sudden changes in nutrition, use of antibiotics, vaccinations, convalescences or sudden weather changes, the use

of Bifidobacteria supplements or Bifidobacteria found in food products can help in the nutritional restoration of the intestinal microflora.

Bifidobacterium longum – is a natural inhabitant of the human intestine. B. longum bacteria are found in the stools of human infants and adults. Together with other Bifidobacteria species, such as B. bifidum and B. longum, they are the predominant bacteria in the large intestine of infants. A separate biotype of B. longum occurs in large numbers in the large intestine of adolescents and adults. They are anaerobic bacteria that produce acetic and lactic acids with small amounts of formic acid from carbohydrates. They ferment a wider range of carbohydrates compared with B. bifidum. The beneficial roles are similar to those of B. bifidum:

1. The prevention of the colonization of the intestines by invading pathogenic bacteria or yeast with which they compete for nutrients and attachment sites
2. The production of organic acids that increase the acidity of the intestines and thereby inhibit undesirable bacteria
3. Assist in nitrogen retention and weight gain in infants
4. The inhibition of bacteria, which can alter nitrates into potentially harmful nitrites
5. The production of B vitamins

If the intestinal microflora are disturbed (and the levels of Bifidobacteria decline) under the influence of antibiotics,

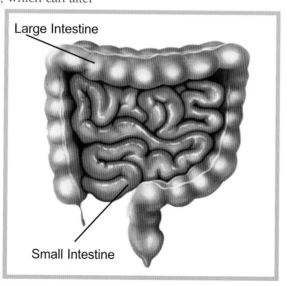

Large Intestine

Small Intestine

8

irradiation of the abdomen with gamma or x-rays, reduced gastric acidity or stress conditions, the use of Bifidobacteria supplements or Bifidobacteria found in food products can help in the nutritional restoration of the intestinal microflora.

A good probiotic formula should contain the resident strains of Lactobacillus acidophilus, Bifidobacterium and Bifidobacterium infantis. Once the bad bacteria are killed, good bacteria must replace it. This is accomplished with a probiotic supplement, preferably one with about four to six billion cultures per capsule. Probiotics should be taken in supplement form during the healing process and after antibiotics.

Cultured Vegetables

In addition to probiotic supplements, another good source of friendly bacteria is raw cultured vegetables. These nutrient-dense fermented foods have been around for centuries. They are rich in Lactobacilli and enzymes, alkaline forming, an excellent source of vitamin C, an effective digestive aid, ideal for pregnant and nursing women, effective in promoting longevity and ideal for appetite control and weight control, as they reduce the cravings for sweets.

Cultured vegetables are 'sauerkraut' (sauer = sour and kraut = greens or plants), not to be confused with the salted, pasteurized variety of sauerkraut sold in supermarkets. The appendix has instructions on how to make cultured vegetables.

Yogurt and kefir (a creamy drink made of fermented cow's milk) are excellent sources of beneficial bacteria. The Resource Directory lists sources of high quality kefir products.

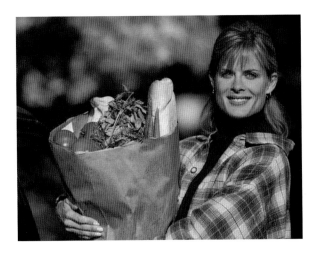

Nutrient Support

Many people believe they can get all the nutrients they need from a 'balanced diet.' Others believe vitamin and mineral supplements are necessary. There's truth to both sides of this issue. Today's produce is seriously lacking in minerals. Consider this quote from U.S. Senate Document #265:

The alarming fact is that food – fruits and vegetables and grains – now being raised on millions of acres of land that no longer contains enough of needed minerals – are starving us no matter how much of them we eat. No man of today can eat enough fruits and vegetables to supply his system with the mineral salts he requires for perfect health because his stomach isn't big enough to hold them...

This document was written in 1936! The situation is even worse today as far as soil erosion is concerned. Between 1950 and 1975, the calcium content in a cup of rice decreased 21%, iron content fell 28.6%, and protein content likewise declined. As nutrients continue to be depleted in the soil, nutritional deficiencies are now the norm, even if the average person makes wise food selections and tries to eat a balanced diet. That would seem to make a case for vitamin and mineral supplements.

> **During your detox/cleansing program for Candida or parasites, it is important to support and help restore the immune system by taking:**
>
> - A vitamin and mineral supplement
> - Additional antioxidants like vitamin C (1,000 mg. twice a day)
> - Essential fatty acids from fish, flax and borage oil
> - Green food formulas for energy

While these may be of some benefit, whole foods are preferred, as they have a broader spectrum of nutrients in them, and their nutrients are more usable by the body than isolated ones found in vitamin and mineral pills. Whole foods contain more than just vitamins and minerals: All the nutrients contained in them haven't even been discovered, much less duplicated. Because of the presence of synergistic nutrients, the vitamins and minerals in whole foods are much

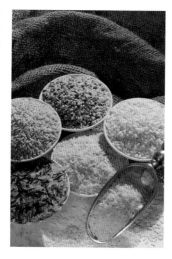

more useful to the body than are isolated synthetic vitamins and minerals. However, since our 'stomachs aren't big enough' to hold all the bulk that it would take to satisfy our nutrient requirements, what are we to do? We have three choices: fresh juices, vitamin and mineral supplements and/or super (green) foods. Juicing is optional, while supplemental nutrients from super foods and/or vitamin/mineral capsules/tablets are a must.

REPAIRING THE INTESTINAL MUCOSA

By now it is clear that many chronic health problems are caused by the entry of toxins into the body, many of them through the lining of the digestive tract. As noted, this lining is called the digestive mucosa or mucosal lining. When this lining is healthy, it will prevent toxins (and parasites, yeasts, etc.) from entering the body. When it is unhealthy, these toxins are allowed to travel freely into the bloodstream, and from there they circulate throughout the body. This condition is called 'leaky gut,' and may lead to many chronic disorders. Therefore, one of the most important things we can do to achieve vibrant health is to repair the mucosa and keep it in a healthy condition. There are some simple steps that can be taken to help heal and maintain this all-important digestive lining.

As stated in previous chapters, the lining of the digestive tract becomes porous as the result of many different factors. Foods to whch we are allergic or sensitive can be either the result or the cause of leaky gut.

Conditions That Indicate The Need for Healing a Leaky Gut

- ADD	- Eczema
- Joint and collagen problems	- Symptoms resembling autism
- Food allergies	- Compromised liver function
- Chronic and rheumatoid arthritis	- Inflammatory bowel disease
- Malnutrition	- Irritable bowel syndrome
- Chronic fatigue	
- Multiple chemical sensitivities	- Symptoms like schizophrenia
- Psoriasis	- Skin disorders (ranging from uticaria to acne and dermatitis)[6]
- Diabetes	
- Fibromyalgia	

Figure 4

8

Some of the other factors noted, which adversely affect the gut lining, are stress, drugs, poor diet, unhealthy lifestyle and the aging process. When the gut lining has eroded, an overabundance of free radical production causes:

- Inflammation
- Irritation
- More leaky gut

This vicious cycle must be broken, starting with the following steps:

- Manage stress more effectively.
- Change eating habits (chew food thoroughly).
- Take enzymes with meals (HCl and plant).
- Make diet modifications.
- Eliminate toxins (general detox).
- Eliminate Candida and/or parasites.
- Take nutrient supplements.

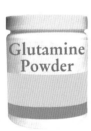

While this may sound like a lot of work, it is a process, not a destination, and patience and trust in the process are required. We do not have to do all of this at once! Between each cleansing and detox program, there is time to work on healing the gut.

If you have any of the problems listed in figure 4, try a program of supplementation that can begin to heal the intestinal lining. Those with neurodegenerative disorders, including senile dementia, Parkinson's disease, multiple sclerosis and Alzheimer's disease may also benefit from such a program.

Nutrients that are needed for the healing of leaky gut include the following:

L-glutamine (or glutamine) – Human studies show that L-glutamine is an essential nutrient for the cells of the small intestine. It is their primary metabolic fuel. Glutamine deficiency has been shown to result in significant functional changes in the gastrointestinal tract. Dietary deficiency of glutamine is associated with atrophy and degeneration of the small intestine. Glutamine supplementation has been shown to prevent and repair damage to the intestinal mucosa due to starvation, injury, infection, immunosuppression, chemotherapy, radiation and chronic alcoholism. Studies show that L-glutamine helps to promote healing of injured gut mucosa. In a double blind human study, 24 of 57 ulcer patients were given 1.6 grams of glutamine per day. After four weeks, 22 of the 24 patients (92%) receiving glutamine showed complete healing based on symptoms and radiographic analysis.[7] Glutamine is a very important nutrient for the healing of leaky gut and should be included in a healing protocol. Dosages range from one gram to 30 grams per day, but the average therapeutic dose is approximately five grams per day. It is best taken in powdered form; taking an equivalent dose in capsule form would not be feasible, as it would require ingestion of too many capsules. L-glutamine has no taste and is easy to take.

N-aceytl-glucosamine (NAG) – is a precursor to glutamine production and is therefore good to take with a glutamine supplement. Human studies show that NAG is a highly active growth promoter for Bifobacterium bifidum.[8] Separate but related 'in vitro' animal studies demonstrate that the presence of NAG can effectively block the adherence of Candida albicans to the gastrointestinal mucosa.[9] NAG is usually included in well formulated powdered glutamine supplements.

Gamma oryzanol – is derived from red rice bran. Gamma oryzanol has anti-inflammatory properties that make it useful in cases of gastritis, ulcers and IBS (irritable bowel syndrome). It normalizes gastric secretions and forms a protective barrier on the mucous lining of the intestines. Clinical studies show that orally administered gamma oryzanol is effective in the treatment of a broad range of gastrointestinal disorders.[10] It has potent antioxidant activity and is a supplement of choice for leaky gut. Double blind studies in Japan showed the effectiveness of gamma oryzanol in treating inflammatory bowel disease (IBD).[11] This ingredient is found in your glutamine powder supplement.

Cranesbill – is an herb with anti-inflammatory properties. This herb is beneficial in an intestinal rebuilding formula as an addition to L-glutamine.

The previously listed ingredients, in combination with marigold (to soothe the digestive tract) and marshmallow (to help rid the bowel of mucus), can be found in preformulated powdered form. In addition to this formula, other substances to take include:

Gamma Linolenic Acid (GLA) – is from borage seed oil and can be effective in the prevention and treatment of gastrointestinal mucosal inflammation. GLA is an essential fatty acid (EFA) that has anti-inflammatory properties. Your daily essential oil formula should contain this EFA.

DGL (deglycyrrhizinated licorice) – usually comes in the form of a chewable tablet that can be taken before meals. It is very soothing to the upper digestive tract and may help promote healing of leaky gut. A good supplement would include DGL, as well as aloe (for its soothing and healing effect) and glutamine (to help repair the gut lining). All of these ingredients are important keys for healing leaky gut.

Notes

[1] Pat Connolly, *The Candida Albicans Yeast-Free Cook Book*, Keats Publishing, 2000, p. 187.

[2] Cherie Calbom and Maureen Keane, *Juicing for Life*, Avery, 1992, p. 87.

[3] Jack Tips, ND, PhD, *Conquer Candida and Restore Your Immune System*, Apple-A-Day Press, 1989, p. 94.

[4] Op. Cit., Calbom and Keane, p. 89.

[5] Ibid., p. 88.

[6] Trent W. Nichols, MD and Nancy Faass, MSW, MPH, *Optimal Nutrition*, Quill, 2000, p. 63.

[7] Amber Ackerman, ND, *Nutritional Management of Intestinal Permeability Defects*,

[8] Ibid.

[9] Ibid.

[10] Ibid.

[11] Ibid.

Chapter Summary

It takes a conscious level of commitment to embark on an advanced cleansing and detox program as described in this chapter. Most people reach this level only when they begin to experience pain. Pain is sometimes our greatest motivator in life. This program has succeeded again and again in clinical practice. When people begin to achieve even small steps in feeling better, they say it is worth the effort. The steps outlined for the advanced parasite/Candida cleanses are designed for maximum efficiency and simplicity. On this program there is no need to fast, take handfuls of pills at frequent intervals or interfere with your normal routine in any way. Anyone using this program will be able to work as usual and carry on normal activities while cleansing. The steps in this advanced cleansing program are:

Diet
• Prepare and plan your meals and snacks for the entire week.
• Have an alternate plan for eating at restaurant, if necessary.
• Follow the anti-Candida diet.
• Drink plenty of water.
• Drink green juices and/or fresh juices, if desired.

Recommended Supplementation

1. Take anti-fungal or anti-parasitic formulas as directed.
2. Take digestive plant enzymes (HCl, if necessary) with meals.
3. Take essential oils (flax, fish, borage), vitamin/mineral/anti-oxidant supplements after meals.
4. Have a green food drink in the afternoon, if needed, for energy, along with a probiotic (friendly bacteria).
5. Take fiber before bed.
6. If constipated, add an herbal colon cleansing formula.

Exercise and breathe deeply
- Use a rebounder regularly or walk daily; breathe deeply while exercising.

Hydrotherapy
- Try colon hydrotherapy at least three times during the cleanse.
- Take a hot therapeutic bath, steam bath or sauna three times a week.

Stay on the detox diet in this chapter for at least three to six months. Return foods to the diet slowly and with caution. Remember: we are working on bringing down inflammation and irritation, so we don't want to put irritating substances into the body. Should inflammation occur, eliminate 'nightshades.' You'll want to drink plenty of water during and after a cleanse (about one half of the body's weight in ounces).

Once the colon has been cleansed, the organs of elimination supported with a general detox and the Candida and parasite issue resolved, it is time to rebuild the digestive tract, with emphasis on repairing the intestinal lining.

At this point, you'll want to continue with items two through six in the supplementation section, while adding the following:

- A chewable DGL/aloe/glutamine supplement before meals
- Powdered glutamine/NAG/gamma orzanol/Cranesbill formula – 1 or more scoops daily on an empty stomach

The basic functions of the digestive system have long been understood. However, the body of scientific information on the intestinal environment and its link to disease and aging continues to grow. It is now known that a healthy, balanced digestive environment is a cornerstone of vibrant health. Conversely, an imbalanced digestive sysem can lead to chronic disease and reduced life expectancy.

As we expand our knowledge of what constitutes a healthy digestive environment, it becomes clear that many of the health problems commonly associated with aging are closely related to an imbalance in the intestinal chemistry and microbial flora. The next step, as practitioners, is to learn how we can better understand the intestinal environment, and how to help our patients achieve longevity and better health through digestive care and a balanced intestinal environment.

Brenda Watson, N.D., C.T., and Leonard Smith, M.D., *The Advanced Guide to Longevity Medicine*

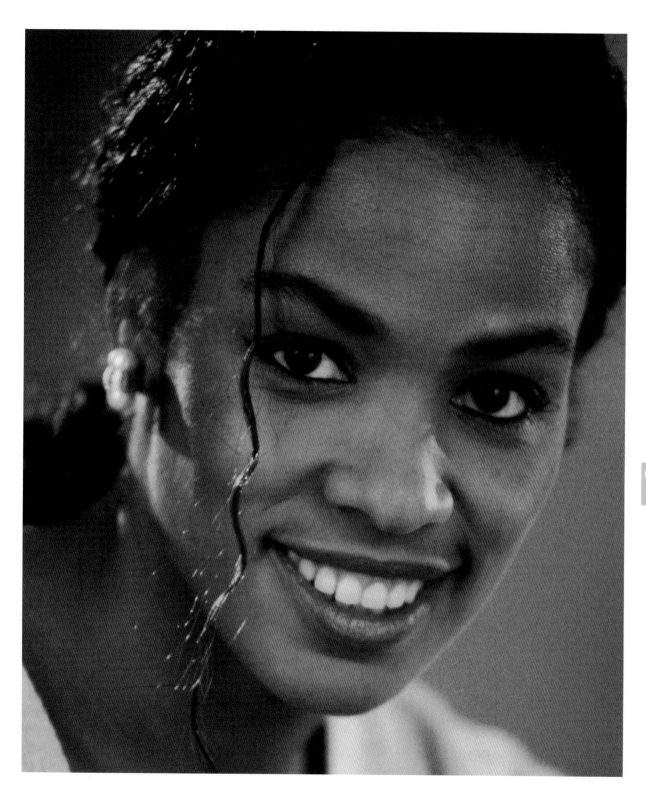

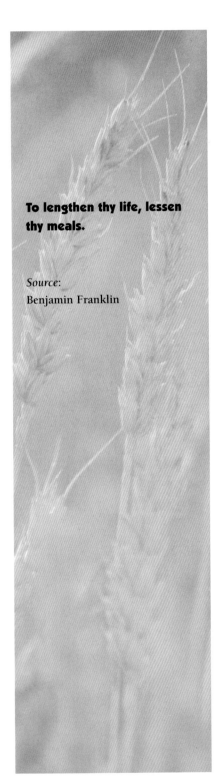

To lengthen thy life, lessen thy meals.

Source:
Benjamin Franklin

CHAPTER 9

LIVER
detoxification
/VIBRANT HEALTH

The liver is the human lifeline. Aging with quality is largely related to the liver's ability to manage toxins. As noted, the assault of toxins in today's world can be, at the very least, overwhelming to most healthy people. For those people who have moved on the Health Continuum (see page 119) towards 'toxic overload,' liver cleansing is a necessity. The number of people today with Hepatitis B and Hepatitis C is staggering. These people need to take a good look at the whole process of detoxification from beginning to end with *liver* detoxification as a major step. The good news is that the liver is very forgiving; it can be restored to optimum levels, and even a damaged liver can often be regenerated.

Who needs to do liver cleansing (which is a step in the Advanced Cleansing protocol)? Everyone! Liver cleansing is important to people regardless of their position on the Health Continuum. It is quite clear why the person in 'toxic overload' should cleanse his or her liver; but it is not so apparent why the person on the 'optimal health' side might may need such a cleanse. For these people, it is important to cleanse the liver as a *preventive* measure, and it is also important for them to include an annual or bi-annual liver cleansing program in their prevention plan. There are several different ways to approach liver cleansing. These include:

• Diet (juicing/adding extra fiber)
• Herbal/antioxidant formulas (30-day program)
• Liver/gallbladder flushes

Diet
A healthy diet should be maintained while on a liver detox program. Such a diet would include:

• Plenty of organic fruits and vegetables
• Fish and organic chicken/eggs
• Juicing (if desired)

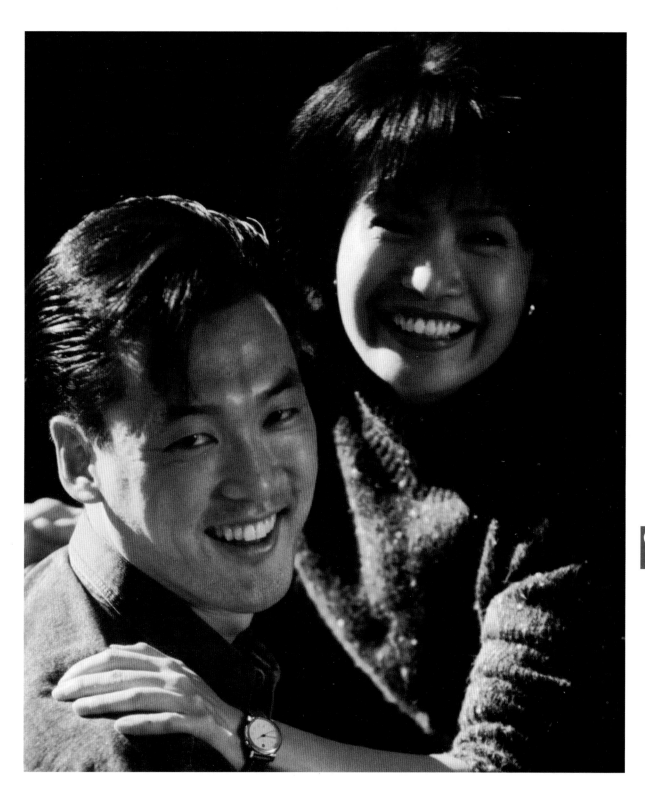

9

- Beets, spinach, carrots, cabbage, cucumbers
- Good oils (especially olive oil and flax oil)
- Water
- Fiber
- Nutrient supplementation

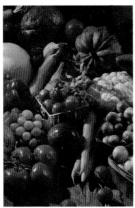

Fruits and vegetables are high in fiber and water. For this reason, it is important to have plenty of both fruits and vegetables in the diet while on a liver cleansing program. Brightly colored foods contain powerful antioxidants that help the liver with the detoxification process. It is important that a portion of the fruits and vegetables be eaten in their raw form, as raw foods contain enzymes that are destroyed by cooking. If the digestive system is weak, however, too much raw food could cause upset. Raw foods therefore should be added to the diet at a pace the body can tolerate. Taking digestive plant enzymes with meals can also aid digestion.

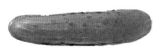

Juicing is always a good choice during a liver detox program. Vegetables like beets, carrots, spinach, kale, cabbage and cucumbers are good for juicing. If juicing is not possible, the liver can still be detoxified and supported through diet and supplementation.

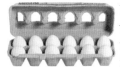

If you're going to eat meat while liver cleansing, it is best to choose organic meat and fish. They are good protein sources, as are eggs. Eggs are wonderful for the liver, with the highest content of lecithin (a fat emulsifier and brain food) of any food. Unfortunately, eggs have gotten a bad rap, although they are really quite good for most people. They are high in cholesterol, but do not raise blood cholesterol levels when the liver is in good health and doing its job as a cholesterol regulator. Eggs are high in the sulfur-bearing amino acids taurine, cysteine and methionine, which are required for the liver to produce bile and generate glutathione, the most important liver enzyme detoxifier. The best way to prepare eggs is poached or soft boiled so as not to destroy the lecithin (a fat emulsifier) content.

Fats and oils, such as flax, olive, sunflower and sesame (that are unrefined or cold-pressed), help the liver build healthy cells. Any of these can be added to salads or taken as a supplement.

It is essential to drink an adequate amount of water (7 to 10 glasses per day) during liver detox. It helps everything work better and is critical for a healthy liver.

Additional fiber, beyond that supplied by fruits, vegetables and whole grains, should be part of a detox program. As the liver is being cleansed, toxins empty into the bile and eventually arrive in the digestive tract. Extra fiber is needed during the detox process to absorb the extra toxic 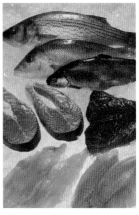 flow. The need for extra fiber will be addressed further in the liver herbal detox program.

Liver Detox Formulas
Liver formulas are usually designed to support liver detoxification mechanisms, while reducing the amount of detoxification stress.

A complete liver detox program would support phase I and phase II detoxification pathways, which are overworked when liver toxicity is present. This support is best achieved with antioxidants and herbs. A complete liver detox program would ideally include three separate supplements:

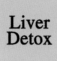

- A 2-part detox system of herbs and antioxidants
- A flax fiber supplement
- Essential oils (flax, fish and borage)

The 2-part liver detox program would be followed for 30 days. Part I would include a combination of the following antioxidants and herbs:

- NAC (N-aceytl-cysteine)
- Alpha lipoic acid
- Selenium
- Vitamin C and E
- Taurine and methionine (amino acids)
- Phosphatidylcholine choline
- Milk thistle, dandelion, green tea and turmeric

This antioxidant liver formula (part I) should be accompanied by a nighttime formula (Part II) that would include herbs

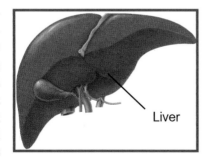

Liver

to increase bile flow. Ayurvedic medicine (from India) uses some wonderful herbs that have been quite successful in liver detoxification. They include:

- Belleric myrobalan fruit (Terminalia bellerica)
- Boerhavia diffusa root and herb

- Eclipta alba root and herb
- Tinospora conrdifolia stem
- Andrographis paniculata leaf
- Picrohiza Kurroa root

Your liver detox program could look like this:

- **A well-planned nutritious diet**
- **Enzymes with meals**
- **Vitamin/mineral supplement after meals**
- **Essential oils after meals**
- **Freshly prepared juice/green drinks, if desired**
- **Plenty of water during the day**
- **Herbal detox capsules morning and night**
- **Flax fiber supplement before bed**

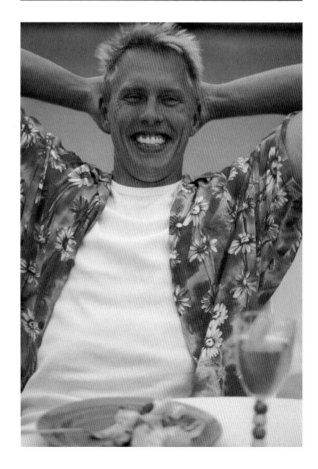

9

This combination of antioxidants and herbs (parts I and II) creates a total liver detox formula, which can be followed continuously while adhering to dietary guidelines.

A good flax fiber supplement added to this program will help absorb the toxins that are being eliminated from the liver.

Nutrient supplementation might include multi-vitamin/mineral support and/or the addition of super foods (such as green drinks), with emphasis on B vitamins.

After completing this detox program, many people feel rejuvenated and have noticeably more energy. Those on the 'optimal health' side of the Health Continuum need this type of detox to stay on that path. Those on the other side, towards 'toxic overload' (especially those with liver damage), need this type of detox as part of their recovery process. The 30-day program may be repeated for optimal results.

Liver/Gallbladder Flushes

Many people attest to the effects of a liver/gallbladder flush even though there is little evidence to support what actually is happening after the flush when round, green-colored, pea-sized masses appear in their bowel eliminations. I have seen this many times in a colon hydrotherapy treatment after a flush. Liver/gallbladder flushes should only be done under the direction of a physician. They are best done during a weekend and must be preceded by a preliminary general detox. One version of many liver/gallbladder flushes includes the following steps:

Monday through Friday – Drink as much organic natural apple juice as possible. Eat normally. Continue to take your usual medications and/or supplements.

Saturday. Eat your lunch as usual. At about 3 p.m. drink one tablespoon Epsom salts in 1/4-cup warm water 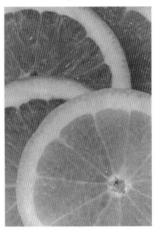 (Epsom salts contain magnesium, which will help dissolve stones). Follow this with freshly squeezed grapefruit or orange juice, to help improve elimination. At 5 p.m. repeat the process – Epsom salts and grapefruit or orange juice afterward, if desired. For dinner, eat citrus fruit or juices (freshly squeezed). Before bed, drink 1/2-cup cold pressed extra virgin olive oil mixed with 1/2-cup lemon juice. In bed, lie on your right side, with knees pulled close to your chest, for half an hour.

Sunday morning – Upon rising (an hour before breakfast), take one tablespoon Epsom salts in warm water. This will help flush the stones out of the liver/gallbladder into the colon. If such stones are present, they will be seen in the toilet with your bowel movement in the form of round greenish masses of various sizes, ranging from small seeds to large 'peas.' Please use caution and physician direction for this flush.[1]

According to Leonard Smith, MD, there are at least a few cases of patients showing clearance of gallstones on their gallbladder ultrasound following a flush such as described above. While stones are sometimes actually found in the feces, it is possible to mistake pieces of fecal material for stones. Dr. Smith cautions that it is possible to flush the gallstones out of the gallbladder into the common bile duct where they could become lodged, requiring endoscopic or surgical intervention.

Heavy Metal Detoxification

As noted in the Candida section in chapter 3, it is necessary to address heavy metal toxicity on the path towards wellness, espe-cially for those experiencing health problems. Heavy metal toxicity must be ruled out for those with chronic Candida problems, especial-ly if they've had a difficult time ridding the body of

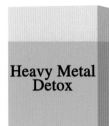

Candida and parasites. Laboratories that test for heavy metals upon practitioner referral are listed in the Resource Directory. The following recom-mendations will prevent metal toxicity or help heal the body while treating it:

- Avoid aluminum-containing anti-perspirants (use natural deodorants).
- Avoid aluminum-containing baking powders (Rumford is okay).
- Use metal-free, biocompatible dental restorations.
- Use non-toxic household cleaners.
- Use least-toxic natural pesticides.
- Use non-toxic cookware (glass or porcelain whenever possible – no aluminum).
- Drink purified water (adding minerals).
- Avoid use of cheap metallic 'costume jewelry' (has a high nickel content).
- Avoid hydrogenated oils (nickel is used in the hydrogenation process).

Heavy metals are not stored in fat like chemicals and pollutants. "They must be pulled from the body by molecular magnets."[2] This process is called chelation (to chelate is 'to claw'). Heavy metals are bound to [held in the claws of] protein complexes of the body such as muscles, tendons and bone.[3] To assist in the release of heavy metals, 'chelating agents' such as vitamins and herbs are used. There are also specific chelating drugs. The administration of such drugs requires supervision of a qualified physician. Chelation with vitamins and minerals can be administered without such medical supervision, using the natural chelating agents contained in a 2-part formula:

Part II consists of capsules containing herbs, sea plants, amino acids and antioxidants. These ingre-dients facilitate the removal of heavy metals (metals that are five times heavier than water) from the body through a chelating process, where the metals are bound to a nutrient (chelating agent).

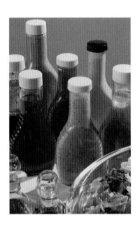

Like many people today, my interest in health was prompted by my personal health problems. I have had hepatitis and Epstein Barr, and faced many other health challenges. It was through the process of detoxification and cleansing that I was able to progress toward vibrant health. The process took about 2-1/2 years. During that time, I changed my diet and cleaned my environment as much as pos-sible. These measures, coupled with natu-ral cleansing and detoxification programs (including colon hydrotherapy), supple-mentation with vitamins and minerals and extra antioxidant support, enabled me to gradually feel better. Today I enjoy a ful-filling life of helping others.

Brenda Watson C.T.

Because of the binding nature of chelating agents, some valuable vitamins (B vitamins) and nutritive minerals (calcium, magnesium) will also be bound and leave the body. These must be replaced. Part I of this formula will replenish these nutrients. Such a 2-part formula includes taking two capsules of part I in the morning and two capsules of part II in the evening every day for 30 days or as many as 90 days, depending on the level of toxicity. It is very important to eliminate all heavy metal sources prior to embarking on this heavy metal cleanse. In addition to key nutritive minerals found in part I of the formula, part II will include:

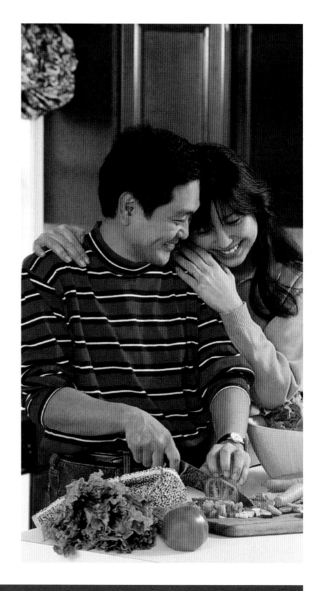

Chlorella – a single-celled green algae that binds to mercury

Cilantro leaf – an herb that mobilizes toxins to move them from the tissue

Sodium alginate – a sea plant used as a chelating agent

Spirulina – algae used as a binding agent

Bladderwrack (seaweed) – chelator, provides immune system support

Garlic bulb – sulfur-forming (sulfur binds to toxic metals)

Kelp (whole plant) – a sea plant used as a chelator

Some of the Signals of Liver Distress Include:

• High blood pressure	• Eczema, acne rosacea, pimples	• Elevated cholesterol
• Chronic fatigue syndrome	• Weight gain	• Brownish spots on the skin (liver spots)
• Pot belly	• Cellulite	• Hot flashes
• Indigestion	• Compromised pancreas	• Abdominal bloating
• Depression	• Irritable bowel syndrome	• Irritability

L-leucine – amino acid binder

N-acetyl-cysteine (NAC) – a building block for glutathione

Alpha lipoic acid – a powerful antioxidant that binds with metals to help move them from the body.

As with other cleansing products, you'll want to use a good fiber supplement while taking a heavy metal cleanse. This will help bind the toxins that are being released in the cleansing process. Once you've successfully completed oral chelation of heavy metals and resolved any oral focal conditions (from such sources as root canals and cavitations), you should feel great!

Vibrant Health

Vibrant health is a goal we all want to reach. To age without the use of pharmaceutical drugs and without pain, depression and fatigue is a goal that should be within everyone's reach. The information in this book has been provided as a roadmap for reaching this goal.

Most people tend to view the detoxification process as a complex one. Simplification is achieved by presenting the process in easy-to-understand steps and using effective formulas designed to achieve specific cleansing goals.

Notes

[1] Elizabeth Lipski, MS, CNN, *Digestive Wellness*, Keats Publishing, 1996, p. 227.

[2] Trent W. Nichols, MD and Nancy Faass, MSW, MPH, *Optimal Digestion*, Quill, an Imprint of Harper Collins Publishers, 2000, p. 256.

[3] Ibid.

Chapter Summary

Liver cleansing can be accomplished through diet (emphasizing added fiber, high water intake and possibly juicing), special herbal cleansing programs (designed to combat free radicals) and liver/gallbladder flushes thought to rid these organs of stones.

Since much of the liver's toxic burden is a result of heavy metal exposure, a special heavy metal herbal cleanse is often appropriate, along with reduction of exposure to these metals. Presence of heavy metals in the body may perpetuate Candida and parasite problems and should be addressed prior to embarking on a Candida/parasite cleanse or if such cleanse has been unproductive.

NSAIDs, such as aspirin, ibuprofen and naproxen, cause gastrointestinal side effects like stomach ulcers and intestinal bleeding. Additionally, they can cause abnormal readings in liver tests. Acetaminophen (Tylenol) can also cause liver problems, which can be severe and even lead to coma and death when the dosage exceeds 10 grams per day. If the person also drinks alcohol, the same damage can occur with only four to five grams of the drug per day. It should be noted, however, that acetaminophen, when taken in recommended doses, does not cause liver test abnormalities.

www.ivillagehealth.com

9

The Health Continuum

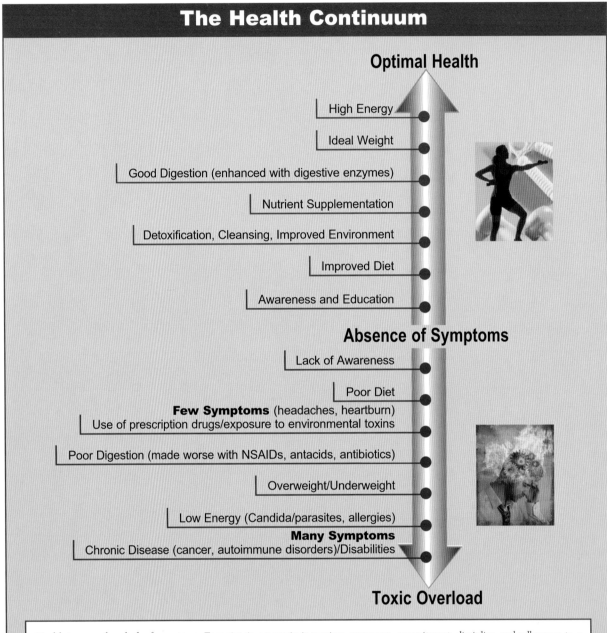

Optimal Health

High Energy

Ideal Weight

Good Digestion (enhanced with digestive enzymes)

Nutrient Supplementation

Detoxification, Cleansing, Improved Environment

Improved Diet

Awareness and Education

Absence of Symptoms

Lack of Awareness

Poor Diet

Few Symptoms (headaches, heartburn)
Use of prescription drugs/exposure to environmental toxins

Poor Digestion (made worse with NSAIDs, antacids, antibiotics)

Overweight/Underweight

Low Energy (Candida/parasites, allergies)

Many Symptoms
Chronic Disease (cancer, autoimmune disorders)/Disabilities

Toxic Overload

Health is more than lack of symptoms. To maintain or regain it requires awareness, commitment, discipline and adherence to a proactive program emphasizing detoxification and rebuilding through diet and supplementation. The net result will be high levels of energy and a sense of well-being.

The road to chronic disease and disability, on the other hand, begins with lack of awareness, poor diet and symptom suppression through use of pharmaceutical drugs. Here the stage is set for the development of digestive dysfunction, which increases the body's toxic load and depletes its energy. The net result is development of more and more symptoms, leading ultimately to degenerative disease.

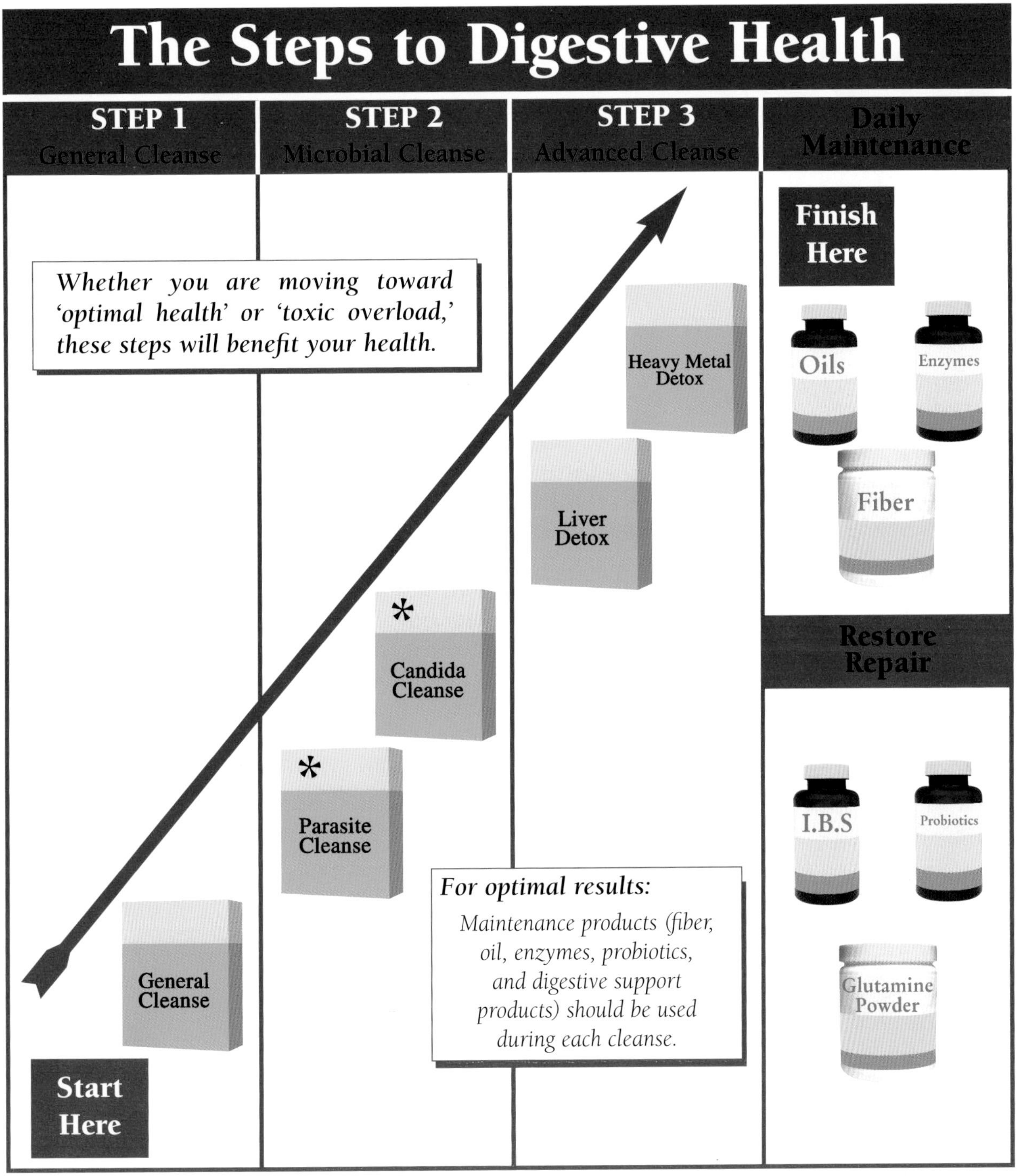

The Steps to Digestive Health

STEP 1 General Cleanse	STEP 2 Microbial Cleanse	STEP 3 Advanced Cleanse	Daily Maintenance

Whether you are moving toward 'optimal health' or 'toxic overload,' these steps will benefit your health.

Finish Here

Oils

Enzymes

Fiber

Heavy Metal Detox

Liver Detox

Restore Repair

* Candida Cleanse

* Parasite Cleanse

I.B.S

Probiotics

For optimal results:

Maintenance products (fiber, oil, enzymes, probiotics, and digestive support products) should be used during each cleanse.

Glutamine Powder

General Cleanse

Start Here

9

* *Those with chronic Candida/parasite problems may need to initiate a heavy metal cleanse (and eliminate/reduce exposure to toxic metals) before they will have success with a Candida/parasite cleanse.*

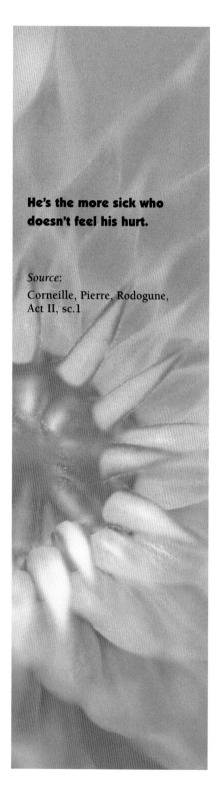

He's the more sick who doesn't feel his hurt.

Source:
Corneille, Pierre, Rodogune,
Act II, sc.1

CHAPTER 10

DIETARY GUIDELINES FOR
health MAINTENANCE

The first step toward improved health is to eat fresh, clean, whole foods – foods in their natural state that have not been commercially processed. Sounds simple enough, but, sadly, eating a 'good diet,' or even knowing just what constitutes one, is not simple at all in today's 'fast food' world.

There are many myths about healthy food selection and preparation. It is the goal of this chapter to dispel some of those myths and describe exactly what constitutes a 'good diet.' Understand that what's being described here is a good *basic* diet, one which will help *prevent*, not treat, disease – though adhering to these dietary principles may well result in the disappearance of some unpleasant symptoms. The 'diet' described here is not really so much a diet as it is a lifestyle, a way of eating. While many may need to begin their journey back to health by following the anti-Candida diet outlined in chapter 8 (which will mean temporary exclusion of some healthy foods), the dietary principles outlined here can form the foundation of a maintenance dietary plan to be followed upon completion of that diet.

You'll recall from Chaper 2 that many causes of impaired digestion have to do with our eating habits – what, how and/or when we eat. In this chaper, we'll look at how to develop healthy eating habits that will aid the digestion process rather than inhibit it.

The components of a healthy diet are organized under these subtopics:

• Time Management and Meal Planning
• Whole Foods vs. Processed Foods
• Balancing Proteins, Starches and Fats
• pH Balancing
• Raw Foods vs. Cooked Foods
• The Importance of Oils, Nuts and Seeds
• The Role of Fiber, Beans, Grains
• Portion Control

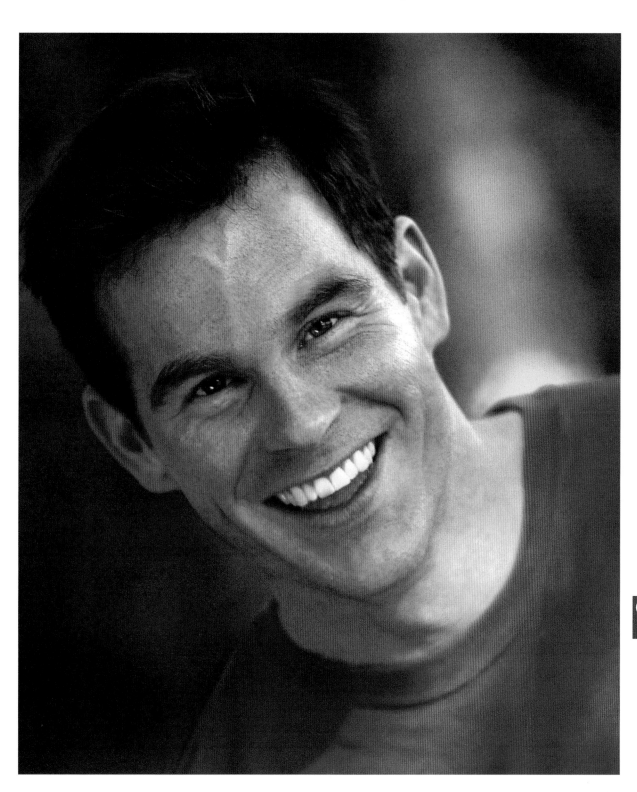

• Vegetarian vs. Non-Vegetarian Diets
• Nutrient Supplementation

Time Management and Meal Planning

Meal planning and time management are key components in creating a healthy eating plan, for food selection is of paramount importance in achieving vibrant health. The first step is reviewing your lifestyle and determining how healthy foods can be integrated into it. Plan your meals for one week before visiting the market. When possible, plan lunches for you and your children ahead of time. Typical school lunches are not very nourishing, and neither are the fast foods so popular at lunch. Ideally, meal planning for the coming week would be done on the weekend or on your day off. Selections would best be written down for better organizing and planning. Make grocery shopping a part of your weekly routine, and make a habit of washing fruits and vegetables thoroughly before storing them. This saves time during the week when time is of the essence. If a weekly plan includes eating at restaurants, then select only those that offer healthy options.

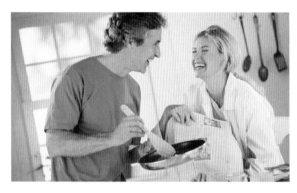

Local markets and health food stores offer the best choices of quality foods to be prepared at home. Look for stores that stock organic fruits, vegetables and meats. You'll want to discard any unhealthy foods – sugar, refined starches, soda pop, etc. – that may have been purchased before starting your healthy diet.

Looking at what you will need in terms of appliances will save you time in the kitchen. One of the most important time-saving appliances is the crock-pot. With it, foods are cooked slowly throughout the day and are ready to serve when you get home from work.

Whole Foods vs. Processed

Any food that is not 'whole' is fragmented, and that fragmentation occurs as the result of food processing procedures designed to extend shelf life and make the food look fresh and attractive. These processes include enriching, homogenizing, flavoring, preserving, milling, pasteurizing, coloring, irradiating, emulsifying, thickening, stabilizing, hydrogenating, etc. While these processes may enhance the appearance of the foods and make them last longer, they do so at the expense of nutrients. Many food processing procedures involve the application of heat, which destroys enzymes, as well as many vitamins and minerals.

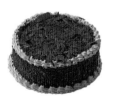 **vs.**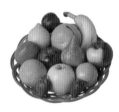

Focusing on fresh fruits and vegetables, preferably organic ones, is recommended when making the transition from processed to whole foods. Agricultural use of pesticides and herbicides has escalated wildly during a relatively brief span of time. Amazingly, as many as 60 cancer-causing pesticides can be legally used to grow most common foods.[1] In 1993, a study conducted by the Environmental Working Group concluded that, by age five, children have consumed more pesticides than considered safe for a lifetime. These pesticides are fat-soluble, so they cannot be washed off the produce (and are retained in the body). Ingesting them puts a tremendous strain on the detoxification systems of the liver. In today's world, it's imperative to 'go organic' to retain or regain health. Washing organic produce in either hydrogen peroxide or a special 'veggie wash' solution is very important, for these foods are apt to carry parasites. Organic dairy and meat products are wise choices as well, since today's 'factory farm' animals are often diseased and loaded with antibiotics and growth hormones.

If fresh organic produce is unavailable, select frozen over canned. It has more nutritional value. Be sure to read labels, and avoid those foods that list chemical preservatives. Also, avoid added sugar and artificial sweeteners, especially Aspartame, sold as 'NutraSweet,® is a "neurotoxic substance that has been associated with numerous health problems including dizziness, visual impairment, severe muscle aches, numbing of extremities, high blood pressure, retinal hemorrhaging, seizures and depression."[2] Other foods to avoid are those containing 'partially hydrogenated vegetable oil.' This man-made oil is found in commercial peanut butter, margarine and most baked goods. Most supermarket oils are refined (unless kept in a special 'health food' section) and not so labeled. Make sure the oil you use is labeled 'unrefined' or 'expeller pressed.'

Most packaged grains found in grocery stores are refined. White rice is an example. Choose brown rice over white. Try some of the less familiar but highly nourishing whole grains like millet, buckwheat, teff, quinoa, amaranth, spelt, bulgur wheat and barley. These are all available, often in bulk form, through natural food stores. You'll want to "go organic" with these foods, as well as others, whenever possible. An organization that has worked diligently to increase awareness about the dangers of pesticides (as well as the hazards of food irradiation and biotechnology) is Food and Water, Inc. at 1-800-EAT-SAFE.

Balancing Proteins, Carbohydrates and Fats

Macronutrients consist of proteins, fats and carbohydrates (simple ones like fruit and 'starchy' ones like grains). Our general health, it seems,

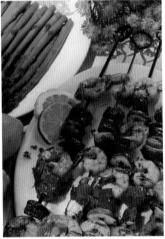

is influenced by the percentage of caloric intake from each of these groups. There is compelling evidence that the high carbohydrate/low fat diet, once touted as the ideal, has some undesirable effects on health: weight gain, hypoglycemia (low blood sugar) and heart disease. Researchers have found that such an eating plan is deficient in essential fatty acids, and the low protein-to-carbohydrate ratio results in excessive insulin release (when carbohydrates are eaten) and inhibition of the hormone **glucagon** (when protein is eaten). The net effect of the high carb/low fat diet is fat storage (weight gain), lowering of blood sugar levels and hormonal imbalances (from essential fatty acid deficiencies).

Dr. Barry Sears, a pioneer researcher in this field, has proposed a solution to this potential problem: the 40/30/30 eating plan (40% of calories from carbohydrates, 30% from protein and 30% from fat). This balanced eating plan avoids the problems associated with the high carbohydrate/low fat diet. However, calculating the percentage of calories from each macronutrient for each meal can be time-consuming and somewhat problematic. A simpler method is to watch (and, if necessary, limit) carbohydrate intake. Also, make sure that the protein food in a meal is about the size of the palm of your hand, and add olive oil to salads.

10

pH Balancing

What's important to know about pH is that most grains, all meats and sugary foods are acid-forming in the body, while most fruits (even citrus) and vegetables are alkaline-forming (though they may be acid in their raw, undigested form). The consensus among experts in the natural health field seems to be that the ideal diet would consist of 80% alkaline-forming foods, 20% acid-forming foods. That means more fruits and vegetables should be eaten than meats and grains. The SAD (Standard American Diet) is backwards, with emphasis on starchy carbohydrates and meat. This imbalance can be corrected by adding fruits and vegetables to the diet while limiting starchy carbohydrates.

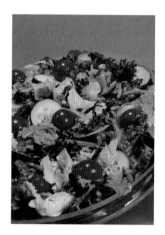

A green salad at least once per day and at least one cooked green vegetable daily, gradually adding more greens, will achieve an ideal diet. In addition to increasing the number of salads and vegetables eaten, you may wish to add green drinks and/or capsules to your daily routine. See Resource Directory for specific products.

Raw Foods vs. Cooked Foods

Chapter 2 emphasized that enzymes are destroyed by 116 degrees or more of heat. Since meats are generally prepared at a temperature of at least 350 degrees and grains at 325 degrees and more, wholesale enzyme destruction occurs when these foods are cooked. Any processed foods, even uncooked, are devoid of enzymes due to the heat applied in the refining process. Freezing and refrigeration also have some effect on enzymes but result in only about a 30% loss.

Enzymes are actually proteins. They consist of amino acids and are the body's building blocks. When enzymes in food are destroyed or reduced, the digestive organs have to work harder to break down and process that food. Metabolic enzymes are then forced to perform this function instead of their intended job of healing. A deficiency of enzymes in the body is synonymous with a deficiency of life force.

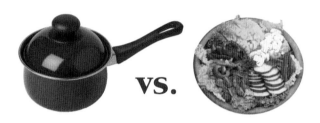

Nothing shows the value of raw foods more than the work done by the late Francis Pottenger, MD. In 1946, he experimented with 900 cats. Half were fed raw milk and raw meat; the other half ate cooked meat and pasteurized (cooked) milk. During a 10-year period, he found that the cats on the raw diet thrived, while those on the cooked food diet showed all the degenerative diseases common in man. By the third generation, all the cats on the processed diet were sterile or congenitally malformed.

Not only do we have more energy (life force) from raw foods in our diet, but our bodies are more thoroughly hydrated due to their high water content. A diet of exclusively cooked foods forces the body to use its own fluids to moisten the ingested food, and therefore has a dehydrating effect. Dehydration is an important, though often overlooked, cause of many disorders including constipation. Those with raw foods in their diet will require less extra water intake than those eating predominantly cooked foods.

Any food prepared at temperatures less than 116 degrees may be considered 'raw.' Although conventional cooking requires much higher temperatures, tasty foods can be prepared at extremely low temperatures or without heat, using kitchen appliances such as juicers, dehydrators, food processors and blenders. There are many fine 'cook' books available at natural foods stores on how to prepare tasty raw foods.

Add raw foods gradually to your diet, especially if your current diet is composed largely of cooked food and/or you suffer from digestive disorders. Some people with inflammatory conditions can't process raw foods, or in some extreme cases, even cooked vegetables. Each person is different and must do what is best for his or her unique body chemistry. The simplest way to add raw foods is to alter cooking methods. As healing of the digestive tract occurs and as tolerance permits, less and less cooked foods are required. For example, the steaming time on vegetables may be gradually reduced so that they're eventually firm instead of soft, or they may be stir-fried to a similar consistency. Vegetables should never be boiled. Experiment to see what you can tolerate. If vegetables are a problem, you may supplement with green drinks or capsules. (See Resource Directory.)

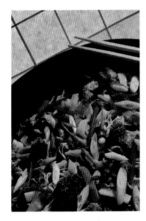

The Importance of Oils, Nuts and Seeds

Oils are actually fats, one of the three macronutrients noted earlier. While people concerned with weight loss are conditioned to view fat as a foe, the truth is that good health and normal weight cannot be maintained without an adequate amount of good quality fat in the diet.

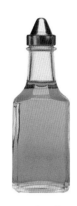

There are three types of fats: **saturated**, **monounsaturated** and **polyunsaturated**. Saturation refers to the way that hydrogen is carried in the fatty acid molecule and to the number of hydrogen bonds in the chemical structure of the fatty acid. Saturated fats include all meat fats, dairy products, palm and coconut oil and the man-made hydrogenated oils. Monounsaturated fatty acids are found in olive oil, canola oil and peanut oil. The polyunsaturates are further divided into the EFAs Omega-3 and Omega-6. The best known sources of the Omega-6s are borage, evening primrose oil and black currant seed oil. Fish oils and flax oil feature a high content of Omega-3 fatty acids.

To maintain health, the body needs a balance of all these types of oil. Problems arise when too much of any given type of fat is consumed. The Western diet has, during the last hundred years, favored fats from meat and dairy products and vegetable seed oils. This has disrupted the balance between Omega-3 and Omega-6 fatty acids. This balance can be restored by eating more Omega-3-rich fats from fish, vegetables, flax oil and walnuts.

Many have heard of the 'dangers' of saturated fat from meat. There is nothing dangerous about saturated fat. This form of fat is needed, but in

> **Fats serve many vital functions in the body. They:**
>
> • **Facilitate oxygen transport**
> • **Lubricate and insulate muscles and organs**
> • **Aid in the absorption of fat-soluble vitamins**
> • **Nourish the skin, mucous membranes and nerves**
> • **Help maintain body temperature**

10

excess it becomes a problem. The same is true of the other natural fats. We've also heard from the media about the detrimental effects of coconut and palm oils. There seems to be no basis for these rumors; in fact, all of the tropical oils contain large amounts of **lauric acid**, which has strong anti-fungal and anti-microbial properties.[3] Furthermore, these oils, like olive oil, have a very high 'flash point,' meaning they can withstand high temperatures without becoming rancid. They are therefore excellent cooking oils. Sesame oil and butter may likewise be used for cooking. While flax is an excellent source of Omega-3, it is very heat-sensitive and so should not come into contact with heat. This is also true of safflower oil, unless it is the 'high oleic' variety. The only fats to avoid totally are the hydrogenated ones and canola oil. Hydrogenated oil is a man-made oil that the body cannot metabolize.

Canola oil has become very popular today, though there has been much controversy surrounding it. Canola oil comes from the rapeseed plant, which has a very high content of erucic acid. Rat studies have found erucic acid to cause fatty degeneration of the heart and other organs. Based on these studies, 'canola' oil was bred as a special strain of **rapeseed** that contains a very low amount of **erucic acid**. Ironically however, it was later found that rats do not metabolize fats and oils well, so that *any* type of oil would be damaging to them.[4] Does this mean then that canola oil may be consumed safely by humans? Maybe not. It seems that this oil is high in sulfur and becomes rancid easily, so that baked goods made with it produce mold quickly. Processed canola oil also contains trans fats, which can be damaging to the body.[5] Considering these findings, it may be wise to just avoid the use of canola oil.

The important things to know about oils are to use unrefined ones and *refrigerate them*. Refrigeration is actually optional for the tropical oils but a neces-sity with other types of oil since they spoil readily when exposed to heat and light. Air exposure will also cause these oils to spoil, so they should be tightly sealed. You will also want to refrigerate nuts and seeds, and, since they contain enzyme inhibitors, which make them difficult to digest, they should be soaked overnight in water to make them more digestible.

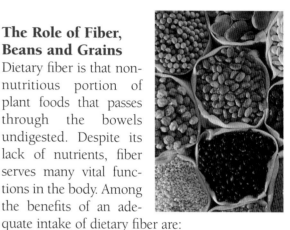

The Role of Fiber, Beans and Grains

Dietary fiber is that non-nutritious portion of plant foods that passes through the bowels undigested. Despite its lack of nutrients, fiber serves many vital functions in the body. Among the benefits of an adequate intake of dietary fiber are:

- Decreases bowel transit time
- Makes stools softer
- Makes bile more soluble and speeds its excretion from the body
- Increases feeling of satiety after eating
- Stabilizes blood sugar levels
- Absorbs toxins
- Reduces levels of cholesterol in the blood
- Increases production of short-chain fatty acids
- Increases stool weight
- Has a beneficial effect on disorders of the bowel
- Increases pancreatic secretion

The value of high fiber diets was first brought to our attention in the 1970s when Dr. Dennis Burkitt published his research on the subject. He noted that Africans eating their traditional diet were not subject to such conditions as diabetes, irritable bowel syndrome, constipation, diverticular disease, colon cancer and heart disease. In contrast, those Africans consuming the SAD suffered from these disorders with the same frequency as Westerners.[6] Dr. Burkitt identified the high fiber content of the indigenous diet as the key factor in disease prevention. There is no question that low fiber diets (like the SAD) lead to digestive disorders as experienced by one out of four Americans.[7] Conversely, high fiber diets not only prevent degenerative disease, but also protect from parasite infestation and actually increase longevity.[8]

Meat, dairy products, sugar and fat contain no fiber. Processing removes most of the fiber from other foods. Since the SAD is composed primarily of all these foods, it's easy to see why Americans are deficient in fiber. Just how deficient are we? We need approximately 30 to 40 grams of fiber in the diet for proper bowel function. Dr. Michael Murray, noted naturopathic physician, researcher and writer, estimated the average daily intake of fiber for Americans to be 20 grams, resulting in a bowel transit time that's more than double what it should be (48 hours, rather than 12-24 hours). Elizabeth Lipski, author of *Digestive Wellness*, calculated a much lower estimate of daily fiber intake of Americans: 12 grams.[9] Of course, Murray printed his estimate in 1993, while Lipski published hers three years later, so conceivably both were accurate. Some

Americans have a bowel transit time as long as *96 hours* due to inadequate intake of both dietary fiber and water.

Fruits and vegetables are high in fiber. So are whole grains and legumes (peas, lentils and beans, except for green beans). When we make these foods our staples, adding good oils, meats and dairy products as 'condiments,' digestion and overall health can be improved. For those on the anti-Candida diet, fruits and some grains, as well as any food allergens, will need to be temporarily avoided.

The fiber present in whole foods is a mixture of soluble and insoluble fiber. **Soluble fiber** is *water*-soluble, meaning that it dissolves in water, forming a thick gel. This gel appears to bind with cholesterol in the digestive tract so that the cholesterol can't be absorbed. Psyllium seed, apple pectin and guar gum are examples of foods high in soluble fiber. Intestinal bacteria ferment soluble fiber into short-chain fatty acids (SCFAs), which have a healing effect on the intestine, providing nourishment to it and preventing cancer. These SCFAs inhibit the growth of yeasts and cancer-causing bacteria in the intestinal tract.[10] **Insoluble fiber**, as its name implies, does not dissolve in water; it is therefore a rougher fiber. (Examples are wheat germ and pure cellulose.) Insoluble

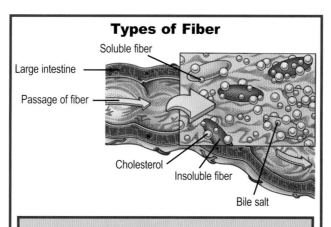

Types of Fiber

Soluble fiber

Large intestine

Passage of fiber

Cholesterol

Insoluble fiber

Bile salt

THE ROLE OF FIBER

Dietary fiber is that component of some foods (whole grains, legumes, vegetables, fruits and nuts) that is not digested or broken down in the GI tract. It adds bulk to the stool and facilitates its speedy passage through the intestine. Fiber helps to control blood sugar levels by delaying sugar absorption. It also binds with cholesterol and bile salts (derived from cholesterol) and may thereby reduce cholesterol levels in the blood.

TYPES OF FIBER

Soluble fiber is partially broken down in the colon. Insoluble fiber passes through the colon without being changed.

10

fiber provides the 'roughage' needed to sweep clean the intestines, inactivating many intestinal toxins[11] and decreasing bowel transit time.

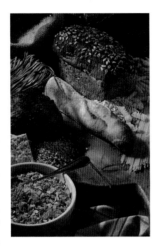

Americans have developed a partial fiber consciousness, it seems. Media advertisements for bulk laxatives (like psyllium) have attracted our attention. As a result, the constipated public is supplementing its diet with this soluble fiber, while continuing to eat refined, low fiber foods. Ironically, the net result is a deepening of the problem, not a solution to it, because psyllium tends to extract water from the intestines, causing dehydration and therefore constipation. There are other problems associated with eating a high level of psyllium fiber: It can encourage "an overgrowth of the normal intestinal bacteria, which deprives the body of vitamin B12 and produces an increase in the concentration of bacterial toxins."[12] Too much psyllium fiber can also increase intestinal permeability and create changes in the internal environment that contribute to the development of stomach or bowel cancer.[13] High fiber foods, such as whole grains, that have not been properly prepared can also be irritating to the GI tract and actually cause damage to the delicate villi in the small intestine, leading to poor absorption. A typical misconception is that fiber is a laxative. Fiber supplements serve as *bulking* agents to push against during peristalsis. Fiber can help to give the bowel movement more form, but it is not a laxative in the traditional sense.

The best way to provide a balance of soluble and insoluble fiber is to eat a variety of fiber-rich foods.

"The best sources of mixed fibers are unrefined cereal grains (oats, brown rice, whole wheat), peas, beans and squash. Among fruits, we get the most fiber per serving from apples and berries."[14] When a fiber supplement is needed, choose one that is balanced in soluble/insoluble fiber. Flax is an excellent fiber choice because it has a more ideal soluble to insoluble fiber ratio.

Proper preparation of whole grains involves soaking them in water for 12 to 24 hours before cooking them. Soaking grains in this manner neutralizes **phytates**, chemical elements that would otherwise prevent proper assimilation of calcium, magnesium, iron and zinc and thus lead to mineral deficiency. Soaking grains before cooking them essentially predigests them so that their nutrients become more bio-available.

Portion Control

Because overeating can put stress on the digestive organs and lead to obesity and disease, many of us would do well to address the issue of portion control. Sometimes the food portions on eating guidelines are not easy to calculate without a scale or measuring device. Therefore, the following guidelines for determining size are suggested:

- **1 ounce of American cheese**
  slightly larger than a standard
  3.5-inch computer diskette

- **3 ounces of cooked lean meat**
  the size of the palm of a woman's hand or the size of a credit card, 1/2-inch thick

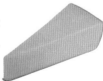

- **1/2 cup of cooked pasta**
  smaller than the base of
  a computer mouse (2 1/2-inch long, 1 1/4-inch high)

- **a 2-inch standard square brownie**
  about the size of a business card

- **a slice of pizza (1/12 of a large pie)**
  should fit inside a standard business envelope

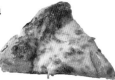

- **2 tablespoons of salad dressing**
  would fill 1/6th of a standard 6-ounce paper cup from the water cooler

- **a 4-ounce bagel**
  about the size of a compact disc

The following list helps to decipher serving sizes often found in food guidelines like the Food Guide Pyramid.' (This information, and the previous, was taken from http://www.thriveonline.aol/nutrition/experts/joan/joan.10-27-98.html):

Bread	one slice
Cereal	1 ounce ready-to-eat
Cooked cereal	1/2 cup
Rice	1/2 cup cooked
Pasta	1/2 cup cooked
Raw, leafy vegetables	1 cup
chopped, raw or cooked	1/2 cup
Vegetable juice	3/4 cup
Whole fruit	one medium
chopped, cooked or canned fruit	1/2 cup
100% fruit juice	3/4 cup
Milk	1 cup
Yogurt	1 cup
Natural cheese	1 1/2 ounces
Processed cheese	2 ounces

Vegetarian vs. Non-Vegetarian Diets

Virtually all *cleansing* diets (except the anti-Candida diet) eliminate meat. During times of cleansing, this difficult-to-digest, fiber-less food is often best replaced by more digestible, high fiber vegetables or by a juice diet with supplemental fiber. While an unsupervised juice diet should not exceed five days, one can safely eliminate meat from the diet for an extended period of time with no ill effects, making for a prolonged cleanse. Improvement in various disorders, including arthritis, kidney disease, skin disorders and gout, have been reported as the result of following a meatless diet. However, many people who have followed strict vegetarian diets and benefited from them initially have found that, after a time, their health declined and did not improve until meat was returned to their diets.

Similarly, the late Weston Price, DDS, found, through his examination of the dental health and lifestyles of a variety of indigenous tribes throughout the world, that the healthiest were those who ate meat. Those primitive people who ate largely grains and legumes were much healthier than 'civilized' people, but developed more dental caries than the primitives who subsisted primarily on meat and fish.

It would appear that in the short run we can thrive on a vegetarian diet; however, in the long run, we need some animal protein, or we risk losing the benefits gained from the cleansing effect of the meatless diet. How long can we thrive on a meatless diet before our health begins to decline? It would appear that the amount of time differs from person to person.

10

There are many factors involved. One appears to be blood type. Much has been written about how people with different blood types have different food tolerances. The point is often made that people with type A blood are inherently low in HCl and therefore do 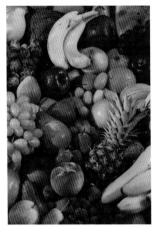 well on a vegetarian diet. What may be more accurate is that people with blood type A need fewer animal products less often than other blood types, and/or that they may be able to subsist more comfortably and longer on a vegan (no animal products) diet than other blood types.

Another factor appears to be the country of origin of one's ancestors. Ancestors coming from 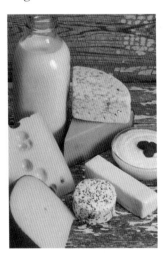 tropical climates subsisted largely on tropical fruits, light meats and vegetables grown above the ground, while those from cold countries lived on heavier meats, stews and root vegetables. It has been demonstrated that people tend to maintain better health when they stick to their indigenous diet than when they deviate from it. Yet another factor in determining the best diet for an individual is the metabolic rate (the rate at which food is converted to energy). Fast metabolizers do well with foods that take longer to digest, while the opposite is true for slow metabolizers.

Regardless of individual biochemical differences, however, it's accurate to say that *most people* need some animal protein in their diet periodically. One person might do well eating red meat frequently, while another can maintain health on bits of raw cheese and egg yolk eaten infrequently. There are many reasons for this. Sally Fallon does an excellent job of outlining these in her section on 'proteins' in *Nourishing Traditions*.[15] The points made below come directly from her book.

It is well known that animal products are the only source of complete protein, meaning that they contain all of the essential amino acids (those not made in the body, which must be supplied through diet). All plant foods are low in three amino acids: tryptophan, cystine and threonine. Legumes and whole grains are the richest sources of non-animal protein, and, when consumed together, provide a complete protein profile (since legumes are high in lysine but low in methionine, and grains are just the reverse: high in methionine and low in lysine).

Many vegetarians eat beans as a primary protein source. While beans are composed of both proteins and carbohydrates, the determining factor as to which of these macronutrients will predominate is the manner in which the beans are cooked. Most cooking methods result in carbohydrate dominance. To obtain the full protein value of beans, they must first be soaked and sprouted, then cooked slowly at less than 200 degrees. A slow cooker or crock-pot works well for this purpose.

Important nutrients supplied in animal fats include the fat-soluble vitamins A and D and vitamins B_6 and B_{12}. Children vitally need these fat-soluble vitamins for their growth and development, which could be adversely affected by a vegan diet. Although the words 'vegan' and 'vege-

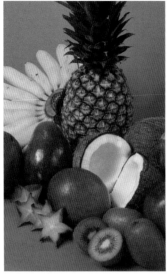

tarian' are being used here interchangeably, this is not technically correct. The vegan diet is a *totally* vegetarian diet, devoid of any animal products. A 'vegetarian' may be vegan in his eating habits, but he *may* also include eggs (ovo-vegetarian) or milk (lacto-vegetarian) or both (ovo/lacto-vegetarian) in his diet.

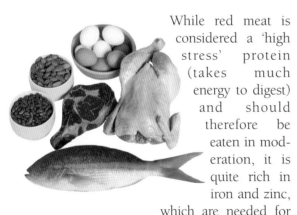

While red meat is considered a 'high stress' protein (takes much energy to digest) and should therefore be eaten in moderation, it is quite rich in iron and zinc, which are needed for the body's use of EFAs. It takes a strong, healthy digestive system (which most of us don't have) to tolerate a high intake of red meat. Once digestive health is restored, however, most people should tolerate it in moderation. Low-stress proteins, such as poultry and fish, are ultimately the best choices.

Although animal products are essential for proper growth and development and for healthy reproduction, it is interesting that "animal studies indicate that animal protein in the amount of one sardine per person per day, combined with protein from grains and pulses [legumes], is generally sufficient to maintain reproduction and adequate growth."[16] This is encouraging for those to whom animal products have little appeal – we don't appear to need much of them in our diet to maintain health. This fact seems to relate to eating habits in the rest of the animal kingdom. Gorillas, considered to be vegetarians,

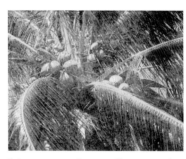

eat insect eggs and larvae, as these adhere to the leaves and fruits on which the animals typically dine. So they are actually eating small amounts of animal protein.

The use of organic meats and dairy products is strongly recommended regardless of a person's choice of animal food – poultry, fish or red meat. As Fallon says of commercial meats, "According to the renowned cancer specialist, Virginia Livingston-Wheeler, most chicken, and nearly half the beef consumed in America today, is cancerous and pathogenic. Her research has convinced her that these cancers are transmissible to man."[17]

Organic meat and dairy products come from animals that have been raised without the use of antibiotics or steroids. To take things a step further, we recommend selection of milk, cheese, butter and meat that is produced from grass-fed rather than grain-fed cows. Virtually all dairy cattle live their entire lives in confinement rather than grazing in pastures as once was the norm. There is a vast difference in the health value of

10

grass-fed vs. grain-fed beef. One major difference is in the ratio of Omega-6 to Omega-3 essential fatty acids. In grain-fed beef, this ratio is quite high, often approaching 20 to 1,[18] (far in excess of the 4 to 1 ratio where health problems start to surface). Grass-fed beef, on the other hand, has about the same ideal Omega-6 to Omega-3 ratio as fish – 3 to 1.

Conjugated linoleic acid (CLA) is a naturally occurring fat that is found in abundance in hoofed animals that eat green grass, but it is greatly diminished in grain-fed animals. Grass-fed animals have three to four times more CLA than their grain-fed counterparts. This is extremely significant, for CLA has been found in animal studies to be highly protective against cancer. Human studies have also shown that CLA helps people to lose body fat while retaining muscle mass.

Unlike grain-fed animals, the grass-grazers have an abundance of fat-soluble vitamins (A & D) in their fat. Also, Dr. Weston Price discovered a fat-soluble factor that he referred to as 'activator X' in butterfat from pastured cows. He found this as yet unidentified factor, which is absent in the fat of grain-fed cattle, to be a "powerful catalyst to mineral absorption."[19] The fat-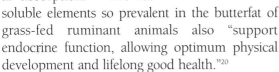soluble elements so prevalent in the butterfat of grass-fed ruminant animals also "support endocrine function, allowing optimum physical development and lifelong good health."[20]

Grass-fed animals live longer, healthier lives than do grain-fed ones. It makes good sense therefore that humans eating products from these healthier animals would also enjoy greater health. There is a grassroots movement away from the industrialization of agriculture back to traditional farming methods. Visit www.westonaprice.com and www.eatwild.com for more information. Also see the Resource Directory in this book.

When completing a cleansing program, animal products will be the last food to be returned to the diet. How much is added and how often it is eaten is strictly a matter of personal choice. The Candida cleanse, of course, is an exception, for the anti-Candida diet does not require the elimination of meat unless you are a vegetarian or vegan.

Vegetarians (and non-vegetarians) may benefit from following the 'Pro Vita Plan' developed by the late herbalist, Stuart Wheelwright, with its heavy emphasis on low stress proteins (that take minimal energy to digest) early in the day. In the Pro Vita breakfast and lunch, five vegetables (one cooked, four raw) and five proteins (one cooked and four raw) are eaten. The raw proteins may be a mix of nuts and seeds (soaked overnight), which can be used in conjunction with a salad or mixed into a blender drink. A typical Pro Vita breakfast or lunch might look like this:

- Salad of Romaine lettuce with onions, carrots, celery, fresh basil, sprouts; dressing of soaked sesame, pumpkin and flax seeds with flax oil or olive oil/lemon/herb
- Broiled cod fish
- Steamed cauliflower

Dinner in this plan would consist of carbohydrates and no protein.

Nutrient Supplementation
While following a prevention program that supports longevity and vibrant health, it is a good idea to supplement with the following nutrients, as it is very difficult to obtain all the needed nutrients from food.

- Plant enzymes with meals
- Essential oils (fish, flax and borage) after meals

- Vitamin, mineral and antioxidant supplements after meals
- Green foods (to alkalinize)
- Extra flax fiber (with borage) before bed
- Acidophilus
    - After antibiotics
    - When traveling
    - During digestive upset (from food)
    - During stressful times

These supplements are great to take everyday. ✳

Notes

[1] Carolyn DeMarco, MD, *Breast Cancer and the Environment*, Health Counselor, vol. 8, no. 6, p. 31.

[2] Sally Fallon, *Nourishing Traditions*, New Trends Publishing, Inc., 1999, p. 51.

[3] Sally Fallon, *Nourishing Traditions*, Promotion Publishing, 1995, p. 17.

[4] Udo Erasmus, *Fats that Heal, Fats that Kill*, Alive Books, 1993, p. 117.

[5] Op. Cit., Fallon, p. 19.

[6] Elizabeth Lipski, *Digestive Wellness*, Keats Publishing, Inc., 1996, p. 159.

[7] Ibid., p. 159.

[8] Leo Galland, MD, *The Four Pillars of Healing*, Random House, 1997, p. 197.

[9] Op. Cit., Lipski, p. 160.

[10] Op. Cit., Galland, p. 196.

[11] Ibid.

[12] Ibid.

[13] Ibid.

[14] Ibid., p. 197.

[15] Sally Fallon, *Nourishing Traditions*, Promotion Publishing, 1995, p. 24-30.

[16] Ibid., p. 28.

[17] Ibid., p.29.

[18] *Journal of Animal Science*, 2000, 78:2849-2855.

[19] Sally Fallon and Mary E. Enig, Ph.D., *Splendor from the Grass*, www.westonaprice.org/farming/splendor.html.

[20] Ibid.

Chapter Summary - Recommended Actions

This chapter has presented general dietary recommendations in the form of foods that help improve digestion and achieve vibrant health. To sum it up, the following list of 'dos' and 'don'ts' combines information from this chapter and others, as well as some new information that will help improve digestion and elimination.

- Choose organically grown fruits and vegetables whenever possible.

- Avoid commercial meats and dairy products. Choose meat and dairy products from animals raised without the use of steroids and antibiotics.

- Avoid commercial eggs. Choose 'fertile' ones, laid by 'free-range' chickens.

- Add mineral-rich sea vegetables, like dulse, kelp, arame to your diet. These are good protein and mineral sources.

- Substitute unrefined for refined oils.

- Assume the squatting posture when having a bowel movement – by propping your feet on a phone book or a 'Life Step™' when eliminating.

- Eliminate margarine. Substitute butter. Cook and bake with it or with coconut oil or olive oil.

- Use flax oil on foods or in blender drinks. Do not apply heat to this oil.

10

- Avoid refined carbohydrates – white sugar and flour products. Use whole grains instead, and minimize their use.

- Favor the gluten-free grains: brown rice, millet, quinoa, amaranth, buckwheat.

- Drink and cook with purified water to which minerals have been added. Do not put tap water in your body. Use a shower filter for showers and baths.

- Avoid canned and bottled juices. Make your own fresh juices – go lightly on the fruit juices; favor vegetable juices.

- Clean your fruits and vegetables (and meats too) by soaking them in a 3% hydrogen peroxide solution in a basin of water, or use a special 'veggie wash' solution.

- Avoid all products containing hydrogenated oils – commercial baked goods, shortenings, margarine, peanut butter and processed cheeses.

- Read labels! Avoid or minimize use of foods with chemical additives.

- Substitute stevia or lo han for other sweeteners.

- Drink an 8-ounce glass of water with lemon juice (to taste) each morning upon rising and each evening before retiring.

- Drink 1/2 ounce of water for every pound of body weight daily (a 100-pound person drinks 50-ounces).

- Eliminate sodas, especially diet sodas.

- Avoid artificial sweeteners.

- Reduce intake of alcohol.

- Stop smoking.

- Reduce or eliminate coffee; use organic brews.

- Use herbal teas freely.

- Never cook in aluminum. Use cast iron, glass or stainless steel.

- Gradually increase the amount of raw foods you eat.

- Soak nuts, seeds, and grains in water overnight.

- Chew well!

- Refrigerate oils and grains – except for coconut oil.

- No deep fat frying.

- Use conventional cooking methods in preference to microwave ovens.

- Eat fruits by themselves.

- Do not combine proteins and starchy carbohydrates at the same meal.

- Use Celtic sea salt instead of table salt (available through the Grain and Salt Society – 1-800-TOP-SALT)

- Avoid or limit the use of commercial dairy products. Select raw milk products if available.

- Don't boil vegetables – steam or stir-fry.

- Limit beverage consumption with meals – They dilute digestive juices.

- Do not overeat.

- Minimize consumption of high-stress proteins (pork, lamb, veal, beef, peanuts, unfermented soy, cow's milk).

- Use a fiber supplement, probiotic and an essential fatty acid supplement with lipase when cleansing.

- Use supplemental enzymes with meals – especially when cooked foods are eaten.

- Try to limit acid-forming foods to 20% of the diet.

- Breathe deeply from the diaphragm.

- Exercise regularly.

- Vacuum pack or freeze leftovers.

Tips for Healthy Living

Eat Your Fruits and Vegetables
Fruits and vegetables are great for snacking. They can calm your craving for sweet or crunchy, plus they are good for you! Fruits and vegetables are excellent sources of fiber, vitamins, minerals and phytonutrients. They can also help prevent diseases such as cancer. Try to eat 5-9 servings a day!

Keep Moving
Incorporate activity into your daily routine. Does this mean going to the gym for an hour each day? No! Keep busy by taking the stairs instead of the elevator, walking instead of taking the bus, leaving your chair to change the TV station instead of using the remote control. Being more active throughout the day may help increase your metabolic rate. An increase in metabolic rate will help you burn more calories during normal day to day activities.

Give Your Food the Attention it Deserves
Take time during meals, and truly taste what you eat. Eat slowly and have meal times be a time of relaxation and enjoyment. Recharge mentally while you refuel physically!

Address Emotions
Eating to soothe your stress is not wise. Try other ways to relax: talk with a friend, take a hot shower, go for a walk.

There is No Such Thing as "Now I've Blown it Completely"
An indulgent treat or a day without exercising is okay. It is better to satisfy a craving than to be consumed by the thought of it. Occasional treats are acceptable – remember that all foods can fit into your eating plan. The guideline for aerobic exercise is 3-5 times per week for 20-60 minutes. Taking a few days off throughout the week is okay!

Tips taken from www.mckinley.uiuc.edu

10

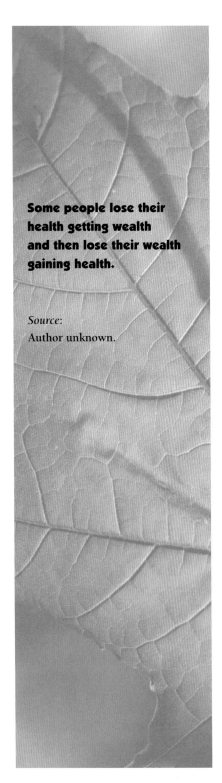

Some people lose their health getting wealth and then lose their wealth gaining health.

Source:
Author unknown.

CHAPTER 11

MANAGING
digestive CONDITIONS

Previous chapters have emphasized how an overstressed liver can pass toxins to other organs of elimination, which themselves then become overloaded and dysfunctional. Consequently, the overload of toxins is carried throughout the body via the bloodstream. The tendency is for these toxins to settle in areas of greatest weakness. Such areas would be *inherent* (inborn) weaknesses or those *acquired* as a result of illness or injury. The net result is that any organ or system can be adversely affected by toxic overload. Those most vulnerable, besides the weakest organs, would be those on the 'front line' – i.e., those organs directly involved with digestion and elimination. This chapter presents some common disorders that can develop when these organs are overloaded with toxins. It also explores some natural ways to support the organs of digestion and elimination when they're under stress.

Digestive Problems Can Affect:

• Stomach	• Small intestine
• Large intestine	• Liver
• Gallbladder	• Pancreas
• Skin	• Lungs
• Kidneys	• Lymph
• Blood	• Endocrine system
• Immune system	• Nervous system
• Circulatory system	• Muscular system

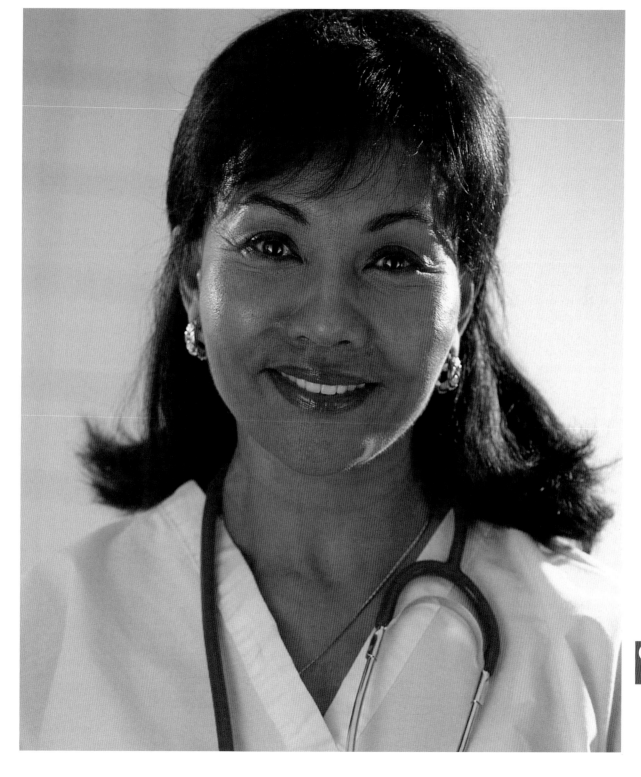

11

Among the disorders that can develop when the body is experiencing toxic overload as a result of faulty digestion, toxic exposure and an over-stressed liver are:

Stomach
- Stomach ulcer
- Gastroesophageal reflux
- Gastritis
- Hiatus hernia
- Vomiting
- Indigestion
- Heartburn
- Dyspepsia
- Nausea
- Bloating/gas

Small Intestine
- Duodenal ulcers
- Celiac disease/sprue
- Food sensitivities
- Malabsorption
- Leaky gut

Large Intestine
- Constipation
- Candida/parasites
- Hemorrhoids
- Diverticulitis
- Colitis
- Autoimmune diseases
- Inflammatory bowel disease
- Diarrhea
- Irritable bowel syndrome
- Crohn's disease
- Dysbiosis
- Leaky gut syndrome
- Rectal itching

Liver
- Hepatitis
- Hemachromatosis
- Cirrhosis

Gall Bladder
- Cholestasis
- Gallstones

Pancreas
- Pancreatic insufficiency
- Pancreatitis
- Diabetes
- Hypoglycemia

Skin
- Psoriasis
- Itching
- Eczema

Lungs
- Asthma
- Bronchitis

Kidneys
- Cystitis
- Kidney stones

Lymph
- Sinus problems
- Swollen lymph nodes
- Ear problems/ infection

Blood
- Leukemia
- Anemia
- Parasites

Endocrine System
- Hormone imbalances
- Prostatitis
- PMS
- Endometriosis
- Low libido
- Infertility

Immune System
- Allergies
- Low immune function
- Cancer
- Environmental sensitivities
- Chronic fatigue

Nervous System
- Depression
- Brain fog
- Parkinson's disease
- Behavioral disorders
- Irritability
- Mood swings
- Headaches

Circulatory system
- Hypertension
- Angina
- Coronary artery disease

Muscular System
- Fibromyalgia

Miscellaneous
- Cataracts
- Arthritis
- Alzheimer's disease
- Macular degeneration

This list is by no means complete, for virtually any condition can develop as the result of toxicity, especially when it is paired with nutritional deficiency. Some of the conditions mentioned above have already been discussed. The remainder of this chapter focuses on those gastrointestinal disorders most prevalent today, as well as on their prevention and non-medical management.

Constipation

There is a vast difference between the medical definition of constipation and the natural healing perspective on the disorder. According to the National Digestive Diseases Information Clearinghouse, "Normal bowel movements may be three times a day or *three times a week...*" The Clearinghouse defines constipation as "the passage of small amounts of hard, dry bowel movement, usually less than three times a week." Here I think there may be some confusion about what is 'normal' and what is 'average.' While the *average* person may have bowel movements within this wide range of frequency, it is certainly not *normal* to eliminate less than once daily. From the natural healing perspective, 'normal' elimination would be at *least* one daily bowel movement – ideally two or three. Since we typically eat three meals per day, three daily bowel movements – one after each meal – makes good sense.

When constipation occurs, food **transit time** (the amount of time it takes for a meal to enter the mouth, then exit the rectum) is greatly reduced. When transit time slows, putrefied material stays in the colon longer, and toxins have more time to enter the bloodstream through the intestinal villi. This can lead to **autointoxication** (a form of self blood poisoning), which causes a wide range of disorders from headaches to autoimmune dysfunction. Additionally, slow transit time can lead to a build up of toxic material on the intestinal walls. This can result in reduced nutrient absorption or malabsorption, which deprives the body of nutrients needed to create energy and vitality. If you complain of fatigue and depression, you could be constipated.

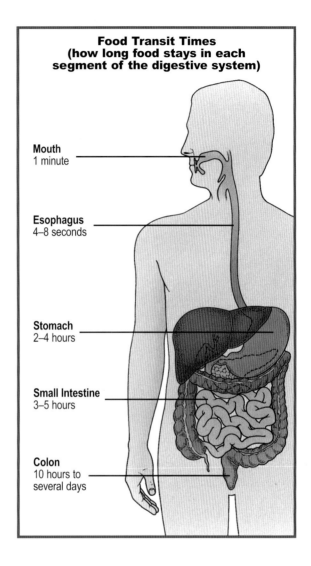

Food Transit Times (how long food stays in each segment of the digestive system)

Mouth
1 minute

Esophagus
4–8 seconds

Stomach
2–4 hours

Small Intestine
3–5 hours

Colon
10 hours to several days

Toxins from food and its digestive by-products can enter the bloodstream when digestion is poor, and bowel movements are infrequent. Once this occurs, these toxins can settle into the tissues, causing many disease states, including autoimmune disorders. Colon cancer, the second leading cause of death in the United States, can result from years of autointoxication. There is a well-established link between constipation and serious disease. The *Lancet*, a prestigious British medical journal, reported in the early 1980s that women who are constipated are four times more

11

likely to develop breast cancer than women who have normal bowel movements.

Constipation is generally the net result of an unwholesome lifestyle composed of many different factors:

Diet: The Standard American Diet (SAD) is made up primarily of C.R.A.P. – that is **C**offee, **R**efined sugar and starch, **A**lcohol and **P**rocessed food. Growing up on such a traditional junk food diet sets the stage for development of constipation. Even for those of us who have improved our diets, the retraining of the elimination system takes time. The SAD is also seriously lacking in essential fatty acids (EFAs). Oils that contain EFAs, like flax, borage and fish, are needed for lubrication of the intestinal system. Sadly, most Americans do not supplement their diets with these essential nutrients.

Lack of Exercise: Exercise stimulates lymph flow, which can help normalize peristalsis, an essential element in producing three daily bowel movements. Our sedentary lifestyles contribute to the constipation epidemic.

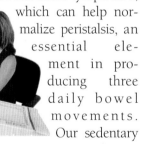

Medications: Many medicines taken on a regular basis can cause constipation. These include antidepressants, pain medications, aluminum-containing antacids and diuretics.

Lack of Time: Repeatedly ignoring the urge to eliminate due to time constraints (having other things to do, which are given priority) can actually suppress the natural urge to eliminate so that eventually the urge becomes less frequent.

Changes in Routine: Interruption of normal daily activities, as in frequent business travel, can result in constipation. Establishing and following a daily routine can help promote good elimination.

You'll recall from chapter 1 that a 'good' bowel movement is one that is walnut brown in color, with a consistency similar to toothpaste, about the length of a banana. The stool would be free of odor, leave the body easily, settle in the toilet water and gently submerge. A stool that is too hard may be the result of insufficient water intake, as well as infrequent eliminations (less than two to three per day). The stool that sinks to the bottom of the toilet is the result of inadequate daily fiber (less than 30 to 40 grams) in the diet. The stool that floats on the surface of the water could be the result either of too much fiber in the diet, or, more than likely, too much undigested fat.

The formula for a good healthy bowel movement is actually quite simple:

Peristalsis: To achieve two to three bowel movements per day, the peristaltic action of the bowel must be regular and vigorous. When peristalsis is functioning normally, food will move through the digestive system in less than 24 hours. **Hydration** is important to normal peristalsis. Though not well known, constipation is often caused by dehydration. The key to hydrating the colon is to drink plenty of water. Hydrating minerals (like magnesium) and gentle, non-laxative herbs, like cape aloe and rhubarb, may also be used to 'jump-start' the peristaltic action of the colon. Cascara sagrada and senna are herbs that are often used either alone or with other herbs to induce peristalsis.

Bulk: The bowel requires bulk or fiber in order for it to move two to three times per day. The right kind of fiber is critical to adding proper bulk. Ideally a daily intake of 30-40 grams of fiber would consist of equal amounts of **soluble** fiber and **insoluble** fiber. This balance occurs naturally in flax-based fiber. Because it is difficult to eat 30–40 grams of fiber per day through diet alone, many people supplement their diets with fiber products. It is important to avoid fibers that 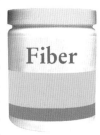 are predominantly soluble, for they can result in dehydration of the colon and subsequent reduction of peristalsis. Psyllium is such a fiber, being mostly soluble. It absorbs 40 times its weight in water. Therefore, it will absorb most of the free water in the colon, leaving it dehydrated and sluggish. This is why so many people become clogged and constipated when they use a psyllium-based fiber product and don't drink enough water. A flax fiber, on the other hand, with its 50/50 balance of soluble/insoluble fiber, gives the user the benefits of toxin absorption and proper bulk in the colon without causing dehydration and the resultant constipation.

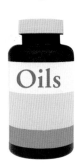

Lubrication: To achieve two to three bowel movements per day, lubrication of the colon is critically important. There are many good oils, including flax, borage and fish, which are very effective in providing necessary lubrication for smooth and gentle elimination. These oils not only provide the colon with the lubrication it needs to eliminate two to three times per day, but they also give the body the essential fatty acids vital to many cellular functions and hence to good health. Because these fats are difficult to digest, it is important to use an oil supplement that includes **lipase**, the digestive enzyme that assists in the breakdown of oils into essential fatty acids.

Following this simple '**PBL**' formula (Peristalsis, Bulk and Lubrication) will result in proper daily elimination. Following the 30-day cleansing program described in chapter 7, will help to satisfy the PBL criteria. The 30-day cleanse is to be used in conjunction with a good fiber product and oil product.

To create an environment conducive to regular elimination, follow these 10 tips:

1. Drink plenty of water (1/2 oz. for every pound of body weight).
2. Change your diet slowly, adding more fruits and vegetables (for bulk), especially organic ones. Supplement daily with a good fiber product. Lower the amount of refined starches, sugar and processed foods you eat.
3. Try taking digestive enzymes with your meals.
4. Exercise! – if not daily, then at least three times per week for 30 minutes.
5. Lubricate the colon by taking essential fatty acids in oils such as fish, borage and flax.
6. When traveling, try to maintain a normal diet and regular sleep schedule.
7. Make the time to go to the bathroom in the morning, even if it means waking up a little earlier than usual.

11

8. Position yourself correctly when using the toilet. Keep the feet raised on a device (such as The Life-STEP™) designed for proper eliminative posture.

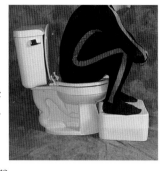

9. Do bi-annual cleanses using herbal combinations designed to support overall body and intestinal detoxification.

10. Use colon hydrotherapy (colonic irrigation) as needed. (See chapter 7.)

While herbal formulas can afford relief from constipation, an alternative method of improving eliminations naturally is use of a warm castor oil pack over the abdomen. The late Edgar Cayce endorsed use of such packs for the purpose of relieving constipation, inflammation and congestion by improving blood and lymph flow to the abdominal organs.

The following are needed to make and use a castor oil pack:

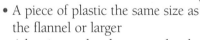

• Castor oil
• A piece of wool (or cotton) flannel cloth large enough to cover the abdomen when folded
• A piece of plastic the same size as the flannel or larger
• A heating pad or hot water bottle
• A large towel

Once you have assembled these items, you can make the pack by thoroughly saturating the flannel with castor oil, and wringing it so it is not dripping. Lie down and apply the pack to the lower abdominal area. Cover the flannel with plastic to protect your clothing and bedding. Then cover the plastic with the towel. Place the heating pad or hot water bottle over the towel, and leave in place for one hour (longer if desired, three hours maximum) while relaxing. Repeat the procedure three times per week or more for a period of three months. Thereafter, the pack may be applied weekly. Following completion of an application, wash the abdomen with a solution of two teaspoons of baking soda dissolved in one quart of water. Your flannel pack may be stored in a plastic bag in the refrigerator when not in use. Add more castor oil to it for subsequent uses.

As a result of normal daily activity, metabolic byproducts such as lactic acid and carbon dioxide can accumulate in muscles causing irritation and weakness. When toxins like indol, phenol, ammonia and histidine build up in the tissues of the intestines, they can be absorbed, resulting in an alteration of the genetic blueprint, DNA/RNA. Adverse systemic effects can result. Eating well and cleansing the colon can help keep the body free of such waste accumulation. So can abdominal massage. The benefits of such massage include:

• Invigoration of abdominal skin tissue
• Promotion of suppleness of muscle tissue
• Stimulation of body fluid circulation
• Balancing of nerve impulse distribution
• Improved relaxation[1]

A form of Asian massage known as Shiatsu has been shown to be effective in increasing abdominal strength and function. The following instructions are provided for this type of massage:

Have the recipient lie face up with the knees bent. Concentrate and enter a peaceful state, wishing well-being upon yourself and the other person. Use the pads of your fingertips and compress gen-

tly but securely, one hand pressing over the other, the points designated in figure 1. Hold each point for at least seven slow, full breaths. Let up slightly on the inhale, press on the exhale. You and your partner should breathe together in rhythm. Breathe fully, allowing each exhale to relax the body and mind more and more. Repeat again at each point...

Follow with European effleurage [stroking movement], using a massage oil or lotion. Place your fingertips just below the navel, pause, then slowly and gracefully begin an outwardly rotating, clockwise spiraling movement. Make about five circular movements, and stop just above the pubic bone. Repeat this at least seven times; better yet 15 or 20. Practice, become graceful with the movements, and spread the health.[2]

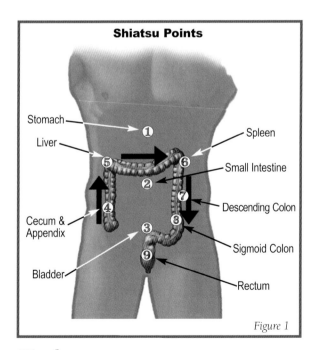

Shiatsu Points

Stomach ① Spleen
Liver ⑤ Small Intestine
② ⑥
④ ⑦
Cecum & Appendix ③ ⑧ Descending Colon
Bladder ⑨ Sigmoid Colon
Rectum

Figure 1

Diarrhea

While constipation occurs when the bowel transit time is too slow, diarrhea occurs when it is too fast. When stool is too quickly eliminated from the body, there is insufficient time for water from it to be re-absorbed into the body. The result is that the stool retains water and becomes runny.

It is important to realize that diarrhea is not, in itself, a disease. It is a symptom. In the case of chronic diarrhea (more than three days), finding the underlying cause is important in determining the proper treatment. There are many possible causes of diarrhea:

- Drugs
- Tainted food or beverages
- Short bowel syndrome
- Cancer
- Fungal infection
- Parasites
- Excess intake of magnesium
- Sorbitol (in excess)
- Fructose (in excess)
- Food allergy
- Diverticular disease
- Malabsorption
- Lactose intolerance
- Laxative
- Bacterial infection
- Viral infection
- Excess intake of vitamin C
- Mannitol (in excess)
- Xylitol (in excess)
- Lactose (in excess)
- Malnutrition
- Surgical resection of the small intestine
- Inflammatory bowel disease (Crohn's disease or ulcerative colitis)
- Inadequate bile secretion (hepatitis or bile duct obstruction)
- Pancreatic insufficiency/pancreatic tumor

Most cases of diarrhea are quite short-lived (acute). They are just the body's self-cleansing mechanism in action or a way of eliminating an irritant. A short-lived case of diarrhea can actually be

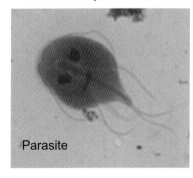

Parasite

11

therapeutic, as it will facilitate the removal of an undesirable substance from the body. People who take diarrhea-suppressing medications when visiting a foreign country can often make the situation worse. By confining the offending pathogen to the gut, it is given the opportunity to multiply and cause more of a problem. Most cases of acute diarrhea are self-limiting (will be resolved without treatment) and should be left to run their course. Medical intervention is indicated, however, if the diarrhea is severe or bloody, and accompanied by significant abdominal or rectal pain, a high fever or signs of dehydration (dry mouth, excessive thirst, weakness, light-headedness). A case of diarrhea in a young child, elderly individual or in someone who is already ill should also be watched carefully. In most cases of acute diarrhea, it is usually sufficient to take the supportive measures listed in the box below.

In case of Acute Diarrhea:

- **Refrain from eating solid food.**
- **Replace water and electrolytes (potassium, sodium, chloride).**
- **Avoid dairy products.**
- **Use a bulking agent (like flax fiber) to improve consistency of the stool.**
- **Re-establish intestinal flora with probiotics.**
- **Take glutamine powder to help with irritation.**

The replacement of electrolytes can be accomplished through use of herbal teas, fruit juices, meat or vegetable broths or special electrolyte replacement (sports) drinks. Dairy products are to be avoided when one has diarrhea because the cells of the small intestine may be temporarily deficient in lactase, the enzyme needed to digest milk sugar (lactose). Replacement of L. acidophilus (two to six billion viable organisms daily) is particularly important if diarrhea has resulted from antibiotic use, as is often the case.

Finding the cause of diarrhea can be difficult for a physician. It may require special lab tests such as microscopic examination and culturing of the stool for infectious agents. Since chronic diarrhea is one of the most common symptoms of food allergy, testing for this should not be overlooked. When a food allergen is ingested, histamine and other allergic compounds from white blood cells known as **mast cells** (in the lining of the intestine) are released. These can have a powerful laxative effect. Where allergy is present, avoiding the offending food initially, then slowly returning it to the diet, is often effective. Digestive aids, such as enzymes and hydrochloric acid can also be helpful.

Where parasites are the cause of diarrhea, they can be treated with a number of natural compounds. Here again, digestive support is indicated, especially the use of enzymes. High doses of pancreatic enzymes and berberine-containing plants such as goldenseal, barberry and Oregon grape are frequently used to treat parasites. "Berberine has shown significant success in the treatment of acute diarrhea in several clinical studies and appears to be effective in treating most common gastrointestinal infections. Its effects are generally comparable to antibiotics and in some cases better."[3]

In acute cases of diarrhea, activated charcoal tablets (available in health food stores) may be of benefit. These may be taken every hour with water, according to directions on the product label, until the diarrhea subsides. Charcoal was used medicinally in ancient Egypt. Over the centuries, it has been used as a highly effective natural adsorbent of gases and toxins in the digestive tract. It therefore can aid in the relief of gas and heartburn, as well as diarrhea. It has also been used as an antidote to poisons and to lower cholesterol. Charcoal should not be taken regularly, however, because it can absorb nutrients and supplements that are beneficial. Do not ingest charcoal tablets within two hours of taking medicines or supplements or take them with meals.

Irritable Bowel Syndrome (IBS)

IBS, once known variously as nervous indigestion, spastic colitis, mucous colitis and functional bowel disease, is an elusive disease. We might call it a 'trash basket diagnosis,' because people who have GI complaints that don't match any specific diagnosis are often told they have the condition. IBS is one of the most common of the gastrointestinal disorders, with an estimated 10-20% of the population suffering from it. Thirty to fifty percent of all referrals to gastroenterologists are people (predominantly women) with IBS symptoms.[4] These symptoms can include:

- Abdominal pain, spasm, distension
- Diarrhea and/or constipation (Usually they alternate.)
- Gas
- Nausea
- Bloating
- Heartburn
- Excessive excretion of mucus in the colon
- Some degree of anxiety or depression
- Bowel urgency or incontinence

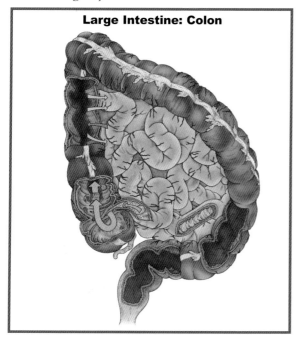

Large Intestine: Colon

- Chest pain
- Difficulty swallowing
- Urinary frequency
- Fatigue
- Depression
- Anxiety

Since there are a number of other diseases that also produce these symptoms, they should be eliminated as possibilities before a diagnosis of IBS is made.

Notable with IBS is the fact that it is strictly a functional disorder, with no identified structural defects. Though IBS sufferers often seek medical help and rarely require hospitalization, the symptoms can significantly interfere with normal daily activities.

Conditions That May Mimic IBS

- Diverticular disease
- Infectious diarrhea
- Inflammatory bowel disease
- Parasites (especially Giardia lamblia)
- Pancreatic insufficiency
- Over-consumption of foods/beverages that interfere with digestion (sugar and caffeine)
- Imbalance of intestinal bacteria
- Celiac disease
- Candidiasis
- Lactose intolerance
- Laxative abuse
- Fecal impaction
- Metabolic disorders such as diabetes, hyperthyroidism or adrenal insufficiency

Specialized lab tests, such as the ELISA ACT or ELISA IgE/IgG4, that pick up various immunoglobins are best used to detect these food sensitivities, which are unlikely to surface on traditional skin tests. Once food allergens are identified, avoidance of all major ones and rotation of all others for a few months is generally recommended. It is sometimes necessary to avoid not just the allergic food but also all foods in the same family.

11

With IBS, as with diarrhea, lactose (milk sugar) intolerance can be an important causative factor. This is a common disorder, affecting 70% of the world's population. The condition is caused by an enzyme deficiency (lactase) rather than a milk allergy. Lipski cites a study where 43% of 242 IBS sufferers had total remission of their symptoms when they excluded dairy products from their diet, and 41% had partial improvement.[5] Avoiding dairy foods for a two-week period can help determine if lactose intolerance is a factor. Whether it's lactose intolerance or food allergy, dairy products can be the cause of the gastric distress experienced by many.

Food sensitivities and allergies appear to play a central role in IBS and are found in 1/2 to 2/3 of those afflicted.[6] The most common allergens are dairy products and grains (especially wheat and corn). Other foods that frequently trigger IBS are coffee, tea, citrus and chocolate.[7]

Lactose is not the only sugar that can cause problems for both IBS sufferers and some with diarrhea. Other foods containing **disaccharides** (two-molecule sugars, which must be split by the body) are a problem for many people. These sugars include maltose and sucrose. Some people have a problem with fruit sugars, in particular citrus fruit. These will cause symptoms (diarrhea, gas, bloating) to be worse. It has also been found that "meals high in refined sugar can contribute to IBS and small intestine bacterial overgrowth by decreasing intestinal motility – the rhythmic contractions of the intestine that propel food through the digestive tract."[8] According to Lipski, infection in the small intestine, as indicated by high levels of methane in hydrogen breath tests, has been found to be an important causative factor in IBS.[9]

Other IBS factors include stress, hormonal changes (women tend to experience IBS before and after their menstrual periods), low fiber diets and infection.

Treatment of IBS involves:

1. Addressing any underlying causes (such as Candida and parasites)
2. Increasing fiber intake
3. Stress reduction
4. Replacement of intestinal flora
5. Elimination of allergenic foods
6. Use of herbs to heal the digestive tract

Herbs can also be used to soothe and heal the GI tract. Studies have indicated that enteric-coated peppermint oil capsules have been "quite beneficial in relieving the symptoms of irritable bowel syndrome."[10] Other nutrients that may be helpful in the management of IBS include slippery elm (a mucilaginous herb that coats and soothes the GI tract), fenugreek seed (an anti-inflammatory herb) and cranberry fruit, which helps prevent kidney stones and bacteria. Also, the *Journal of the American Medical Association* makes reference to a specific combination of Chinese herbs, which has been shown to effectively treat IBS.[11] I have used this herbal combination and the aforementioned herbs in a formula designed to soothe the symptoms associated with IBS. Product inserts have information about specific products that contain this combination of Chinese herbs.

Those IBS sufferers who experience constipation may benefit from the use of castor oil packs as described in the section on constipation. Such packs are also beneficial to liver function.

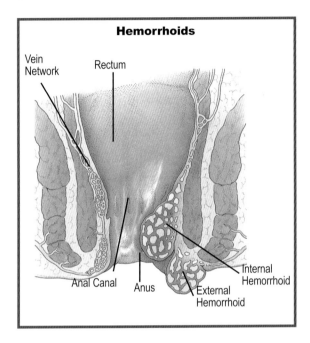

Hemorrhoids

Vein Network

Rectum

Anal Canal

Anus

Internal Hemorrhoid

External Hemorrhoid

Hemorrhoids

Hemorrhoids or piles are dilations of veins in the anal area, either internal or external to the anal canal. These enlarged blood vessels are similar to varicose veins in that they swell and stretch under pressure. Symptoms of hemorrhoids include pain, itching, burning, swelling and possible bleeding or blood in the stool and prolapse. Causes may include:

- Genetic weakness of veins
- Constipation
- Diarrhea
- Pregnancy
- Prolonged standing or sitting
- Heavy lifting
- Vitamin deficiencies (especially B vitamins)
- Aging

Hemorrhoids are extremely common in the U.S., affecting 50% of people older than 50 years of age and as much as 1/3 of the total population.[12] While common in this country, the condition is rarely seen in those cultures consuming high fiber, unrefined foods.[13] Lack of fiber causes one to strain during bowel movements in an effort to pass small, hard, dehydrated stools. The effect of such straining is an increase in abdominal pressure, which results in obstruction of blood flow through the veins, significantly weakening them.

The medical approach to treating uncomplicated hemorrhoids consists primarily of warm sitz baths (a partial-immersion bath of the pelvic area), use of medicinal suppositories or ointments and supplemental fiber (often a psyllium-based product such as Metamucil®). For more serious cases, surgery may be performed. It should be noted that over-the-counter suppositories may contain potentially harmful ingredients. Preparation H, for example, contains mercury and therefore should not be used for prolonged periods[14] or by mercury-toxic individuals, as this metal is readily absorbed through the anal canal.

As with most disorders, the best approach to hemorrhoids is prevention. Straining with bowel movements should be avoided, as well as sitting or standing for long periods of time. Sufficient dietary fiber will help to maintain normal eliminations. This translates into eating lots of whole foods – fruits, vegetables and whole grains – and using supplemental fiber (preferably flax) when needed. It is also critically important to drink a sufficient amount of water daily. Use herbal formulas and/or castor oil packs to combat constipation when necessary.

11

When hemorrhoids do develop, there are a variety of natural ways to treat the condition. **Flavonoids**, a group of plant pigments that have been shown to protect against heart disease, cancer and strokes, can help by strengthening veins. These flavonoids include rutin and citrus bioflavonoid preparations. Of particular benefit are hydroxyethylrutosides (**HER**), shown in a double-blind study to relieve the symptoms of 90% of subjects (when taken at doses of 100 mg. daily for four weeks), compared to only 12% of a placebo group.[15]

Of even greater proven benefit are glycosaminoglycans (**GAGs**), structural components vital to healthy blood vessels. Drs. Michael Murray and Joseph Pizzorno state that "a mixture of highly purified bovine-derived GAGs that are also naturally present in the human aorta...has been shown to protect and promote normal artery and vein function.[16] They cite two double-blind studies demonstrating that GAGs at a dose of 72 mg. per day were far more effective than either HER or bilberry (a flavonoid-rich herb) extract in the treatment of hemorrhoids and varicose veins.

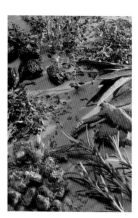

There is a variety of other herbs, such as butcher's broom, which are useful in the treatment of hemorrhoids. In our experience, the most effective is an Indian herbal formula that dates to the practices of Hindu physicians some 4000 years ago. Pilex® is a patented dietary supplement containing three herbs (neem, nagkesar and barberry), which have been used widely in Ayuredic medicine. The formula comes in capsule form and is taken one per day orally for 7 consecutive days. For chronic cases, recommended doses are somewhat higher. Amazingly, this simple protocol has been shown to offer as much as six months relief from the pain, itching, burning and bleeding associated with hemorrhoids. As physician's reports and patient testimonials indicate (see www.varicose.com), Pilex® stops the bleeding and shrinks inflammation, sometimes obviating the need for surgical intervention. See our Resource Directory for information on how to contact the company.

The hemorrhoid sufferer will want to avoid straining when evacuating the bowel. Assuming the natural squatting posture 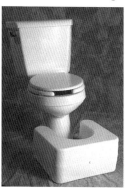 during eliminations will assist toward this end. As noted previously, the squatting posture can be simulated by raising the feet while sitting on the toilet, resting them on a stack of books or on a LifeSTEP™, a device designed specifically for this purpose. The LifeSTEP™ is very effective and can be easily cleaned.

Heartburn

The most common causes of heartburn are food-related (what is eaten and how it's eaten), as is the case with most other problems of the digestive tract! These food-related issues can include:

Overeating – can cause pressure in the stomach, which may result in stomach contents backing into the esophagus creating heartburn. Portion control is very important in managing heartburn. Most people consume more food in one meal than the stomach can digest. Smaller meals eaten more frequently are best.

Drinking too much liquid with meals – Drinking too much water or other beverages with meals can create problems. Any beverage can dilute enzymes and cause indigestion when taken with meals.

Eating too fast – Food that enters the stomach in large chunks does not break down easily. Also, when food is eaten too quickly, the stomach becomes distended, and food is pushed against the top of it where it can intrude into the esophagus. This reflux of gastric contents can cause heartburn.

Too many fatty (and fried) foods – Ingestion of fatty foods prolongs the time it takes the stomach to empty by decreasing peristalsis and lowering gastric tone.

Too much alcohol can irritate the lining of the esophagus.

Other factors that may contribute to heartburn include:

• Pregnancy
• Smoking
• Overweight
• Food allergies
• Drugs
• Infection (caused by H. pylori)
• Too much or too little stomach acid
• Constipation

Supplementation and diet guidelines for heartburn are listed below:

1. Rule out H-pylori infection. (See your doctor for this.)
2. People with low stomach acid are advised to take HCl supplements. These should be taken after meals to see if symptoms are reduced. If you feel a burning sensation in the stomach, then you probably make enough acid, and a supplement is unnecessary. The burning can be neutralized with a combination of baking soda and water or milk.
3. Digestive enzymes from plants work well in the stomach. Plant enzymes are not affected by stomach acid and have protease, amylase and lipase for digestion of protein, starch and fat. A good enzyme supplement would include soothing ingredients like ginger, marshmallow and gamma oryzanol.
4. DGL (deglycyrrhizinated licorice), aloe and glutamine, a chewable supplement, taken before a meal, can also soothe the stomach.
5. Probiotics, like acidophilus and bifidus, help establish and maintain proper bacterial balance in the intestines.
6. Meals should be smaller and more frequent.
7. Drink plenty of water (between meals).
8. Start a detoxification and cleansing program as soon as possible.

Peptic Ulcers
As earlier stated, ulcers are most likely due to the bacteria H. pylori. For many years it was thought that they were the result of stress and high levels of stomach acid. An Australian doctor, Barry Marshall, discovered H. pylori to be the main cause of ulcers. This bacterium must be eliminated before the ulcer will heal. If H. pylori is diagnosed, it is treated by physicians with an antibiotic, an anti-parasitic drug, an H2 blocker, (blocks production of stomach acid) and bismuth. This is ideally a short-term therapy, for problems can result when H2 blockers are taken over a long period of time. The prolonged use of antacids can adversely affect digestion (especially of protein) and create a myriad of other problems in

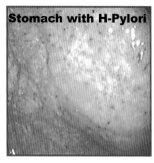

Stomach with H-Pylori

the body by promoting the overgrowth of bacteria and fungus in the stomach and leading to intestinal toxemia. Most of the time, if this short-term treatment plan is accompanied with diet and lifestyle changes, health can be restored.

In the acute phase of ulcers, the following could be helpful:

- If the pain is acute, take some baking soda and water.
- Take one to two table-spoons of either aloe

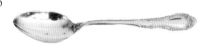

vera juice or chlorophyll in a glass of water.
- Drink plain water (four to six glasses) at the onset of pain to dilute stomach acid.

After H. pylori has been eliminated or determined not to be present, the following natural approaches may be helpful:

- Supplement with antioxidants like zinc, vitamins A, C and B6.
- A chewable DGL supplement (with aloe and glutamine), as described in the gastritis section, can be used.
- Add an extra fiber supplement. A flax formula enhanced with slippery elm, marshmallow and glutamine would be beneficial.
- Add an essential oil formula of flax, fish and borage with lipase enzyme.
- Change eating habits to exclude coffee, tea, fried foods, sugar, refined carbohydrates, alcohol and tobacco.

- Reduce the amount of meat in the diet. Go on the anti-Candida diet outlined in Chapter 8.
- Stop taking NSAIDS (Ibuprofen, aspirin, Tylenol).
- Once healing has occurred, begin a detoxification and cleansing program as outlined in this book.
- Use L-glutamine to rebuild the mucosal lining that protects the stomach. This can speed the recovery time for healing the stomach or duodenum lining.

INFLAMMATION

Any part of the digestive tract can become irritated or inflamed. When it does, it is called an 'itis.' Esophag**itis** is inflammation of the esophagus. Gastr**itis** is inflammation of the stomach. Enter**itis** is the inflammation of the small intestine. Ile**itis** is inflammation of the last part of the small intestine. Col**itis** is the inflammation of the colon. Proct**itis** is the inflammation of the rectum. The next section presents a few of the 'itises' (inflammation) of the digestive tract and suggests some natural ways to help these inflamed organs. Since most problems of the digestive tract are the result of lifestyle and diet, it is necessary to initiate change in these areas so healing can occur.

Gastritis

Gastritis is inflammation of the stomach. Inflammation can occur with or without ulceration. Some of the common causes of gastritis are:

- Medications: cortisone drugs, NSAIDS, antibiotics, cancer drugs
- Alcohol
- Severe stress
- Low HCl production

Some natural solutions for gastritis include:

- Consume large amounts of water. Drinking four to six glasses of water at the onset of pain can help reduce or eliminate it, according to Dr. Batmanghelidj, author of *Your Body's Many Cries for Water*.

- DGL (deglycyrrhizinated licorice) helps heal the mucosal lining of the stomach and increase the blood flow to the stomach.
- Glutamine is very soothing and healing to the mucous lining of the stomach. It is fuel for the cells of the lining of the stomach.
- Aloe is soothing and healing to the mucous lining of the stomach. A chewable DGL, glutamine and aloe combination can be taken before the meals to soothe the stomach.
- A powdered glutamine supplement enhanced with gamma oryzanol can help relieve symptoms of gastritis. Take this powder on an empty stomach to help support the mucous lining of the stomach when irritation occurs.
- An essential fatty acid supplement with flax, fish and borage oils and the enzyme lipase for better digestion of the oils is helpful.
- Once healing is complete, start a detoxification and cleansing program.

Colitis

Colitis is inflammation of the colon, which starts in the rectum and moves through the colon. Symptoms usually include:

- Diarrhea
- Sharp abdominal pain
- Rectal bleeding
- Frequent and urgent elimination during the day (sometimes right after eating)

Colitis can be mild (with few symptoms), moderate (with mucus in the stool) or severe (with blood and mucus in the stool). Traditionally, ulcerative colitis is characterized by blood in the stool, abdominal pain and diarrhea. It is advisable to check for yeast if you have colitis. Complete the Candida questionnaire in the appendix.

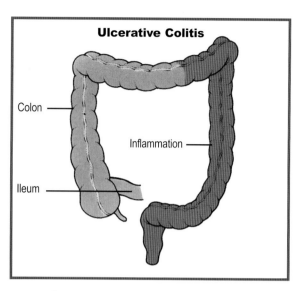

Most digestive problems are due to poor diet. This is also true for colitis. The foods that contribute to colitis are:

- Low fiber foods
- Too much sugar and refined carbohydrates
- Dairy products
- Too little fruits and vegetables
- Food allergens

Some suggestions for managing colitis naturally include:

- Go on the anti-Candida diet (see Chapter 8), abstaining from wheat, dairy and sugar. Stay on this diet until your body has healed, regardless of the severity of your condition. Avoid raw foods when the stools are loose. Choose steamed vegetables, as they are easier to digest.
- Add green drinks (no fruit) after loose stools have stopped. The Resource Directory has a listing of green supplements.
- Take a fiber supplement like flax combined with slippery elm, marshmallow and glutamine.
- Supplement with glutamine powder containing gamma oryzanol, ginger and cranesbill.
- Take an essential oil supplement containing flax, fish and borage oils with added lipase.

11

- Add an extra fish oil supplement (3,000 mg. EPA and 2,000 mg. DHA per day).
- Take a probiotic supplement containing acidophilus and bifidus (six billion cultures per cap), two capsules twice a day.
- Take extra zinc and vitamins C and A for antioxidant support.

Start the anti-Candida diet, and stay on it for a week before starting the supplement program. (Go slowly, if necessary, one supplement every day or two.) Begin with the glutamine, fish oils and probiotics. Add antioxidant support and essential oils last.

Colon hydrotherapy is indicated for mild to moderate colitis. It is contraindicated for ulcerative colitis.

After healing, try a detox and cleansing program.

Diverticular Conditions

The colon is a five feet long tube lined on the inside with smooth muscle. This muscle contracts (peristalsis) to expel waste. Most people think the colon looks like the pictures in anatomy/physiology books – round and healthy. People living on the SAD (Standard American Diet), which is low in fiber and high in fat and sugar, can have narrow, pocketed, inflamed areas in the colon. As we age, this organ deteriorates slowly (and often silently), and before we know it, we have developed some type of health problem caused by a colon that is distorted beyond recognition.

Diverticula occur when the colon forms pockets from the inside out. These little pockets can develop throughout the colon. Most of the time they are concentrated on the left side or sigmoid portion of the colon. Constipation can also accompany diverticular problems due to pressure in the colon.

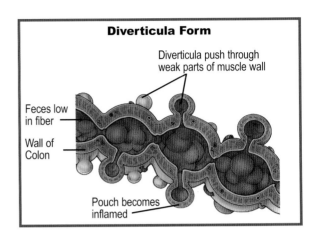

Some people with diverticular problems are asymptomatic (without symptoms); others have some pain and tenderness, even spasticity with diverticular pocketing. These diverticular sacs often harbor bad bacteria, causing infection known as **diverticulitis**. Once diverticulitis occurs, it usually is treated with antibiotics or surgery. A person who develops diverticulitis is in pain and should be checked by a physician.

To manage the condition of diverticular pocketing:

- Add more fiber to the diet in the form of:
  Beans (properly soaked and cooked)
  Grains (not boxed cereals), soaked overnight
  Vegetables (raw and cooked) – Remember to chew, chew and chew.

- Take supplements:
  Flax fiber (powder or capsules) – such fiber, formulated with combinations of slippery elm and marshmallow, will soothe the irritated colon.
  Essential oils – flax, fish, borage with the digestive enzyme lipase in a gel capsule to help break down fat and support the digestive tract
  Probiotics – like acidophilus and bifidus (six billion cultures per capsule at time of manufacture), plus ginger, marshmallow, papaya and bromelain

Plant enzymes with meals – to include protease, amylase and lipase for digestion of protein and fat

A detox and cleansing program with herbs and colon hydrotherapy should be a part of a prevention program for anyone with diverticular conditions. Chapter 7 has the details. ❋

Notes

1 Joseph Vargas, PhD., "Abdominal Massage," *ACTA Quarterly*, fall, 1992, p. 35.

2 Ibid.

3 Michael Murray ND and Joseph Pizzorno, ND, *Encyclopedia of Natural Medicine*, Prima Health, 1998, p. 437.

4 Ibid., p. 609.

5 Elizabeth Lipski, *Digestive Wellness*, Keats Publishing, Inc., 1996, pgs. 238-239.

6 Ibid., pg 238.

7 Ibid.

8 Op. Cit., Murray and Pizzorno, p. 611.

9 Op. Cit., Lipski, p. 239.

10 Op. Cit., Murray and Pizzorno, p. 611.

11 *Journal of the American Medical Association*, 1998 November 11; 280 (18): 1585-9.

12 Op. Cit., Murray and Pizzorno, p. 507.

13 Ibid., p. 508

14 Trent W. Nichols, MD and Nancy Faass, MSW, MPH, *Optimal Digestion*, Quill, 1999, p. 550.

15 Op. Cit., Murray and Pizzorno, p. 510.

16 Ibid.

Fiber Content of Foods

Apple	1 medium	=	4 grams
Peach	1 medium	=	2 grams
Pear	1 medium	=	4 grams
Acorn squash, fresh, cooked	3/4 cup	=	7 grams
Broccoli, fresh, cooked	1/2 cup	=	2 grams
Zucchini, fresh, cooked	1 cup	=	2.5 grams
Brown rice, cooked	1 cup	=	3.5 grams
Cereal, bran flakes	3/4 cup	=	5 grams
Oatmeal, plain, cooked	3/4 cup	=	3 grams

Source: www.nal.usda.gov/fnic/cgi/nut_search.pl

Chapter Summary

Disease is the result of toxicity and nutrient deficiency. Virtually any disease can be caused from toxic build up in the body when the liver is over-burdened.

Constipation can be avoided or corrected by assuring that the bowel is sufficiently hydrated, has adequate bulk and is lubricated with EFA-rich oil. Herbal formulas and castor oil packs can help relieve constipation.

While most acute cases of diarrhea are self-limiting and actually assist the body in its cleansing process, chronic cases may be a sign of serious illness. Irritable bowel syndrome, an ill-defined set of GI symptoms, generally responds well to herbal therapy and dietary management, as does heartburn, peptic ulcers, diverticular conditions and those involving inflammation, such as colitis and gastritis.

Hemorrhoids can be prevented by keeping water and fiber content high. Some herbal and other natural remedies afford impressive relief.

Most digestive problems are due to poor diet (low in fiber, high in sugar and allergens) and inadequate water intake. They generally respond well to improved diet, increased water intake and use of appropriate supplements. The basics are flax fiber, EFAs, probiotics and plant enzymes.

11

CHAPTER 12

children

In 12 children (mean age of 58 1/4 months, males) who had severe constipation of 3 or fewer stools per week, the elimination of cow's milk protein resulted in a dramatic improvement in constipation symptoms.

Source:
Clinical Pearls News, April 2002

The strongest impulse most adults feel, after their own individual survival instinct, is the impulse to help their children, to keep them safe and healthy. This is becoming an increasingly difficult task in today's toxic world where physical and mental illness are escalating rapidly.

Our children are growing up in a much more toxic environment than we did. Increases in the toxicity of food, water and air place our children at considerable physical risk. Much of today's farm produce looks good but doesn't have the nutritional value children (and adults) need. The net result of demineralization of the soil, processing of foods and widespread use of chemical fertilizers, pesticides and herbicides is devitalized, toxic food that cannot create or support good health.

To this physical stress is added the emotional stress of today's fast-paced society. Most children today are raised either in single-parent households or in two income families. The effect is stressful for all concerned. The child in these circumstances internalizes much of that stress. Emotional stress, combined with increased environmental toxicity and inadequate nutrition, can cause a significant weakening of a child's normally strong and resilient immune system. This can result in ear or throat infections, flu and other common childhood illnesses that typically cause the worried parent and sick child to visit the doctor's office. All too often, the treatment of choice, following a cursory examination, is a broad-spectrum antibiotic. Such treatment can have the net effect of depressing immunity by killing good as well as bad bacteria in the gut, allowing for the proliferation of opportunistic infections such as Candida and parasites. In this chapter, we'll look at nonmedical ways to manage these conditions in children, as well as focus on two of today's most widespread childhood disorders – earaches and Attention Deficit Disorder (ADD).

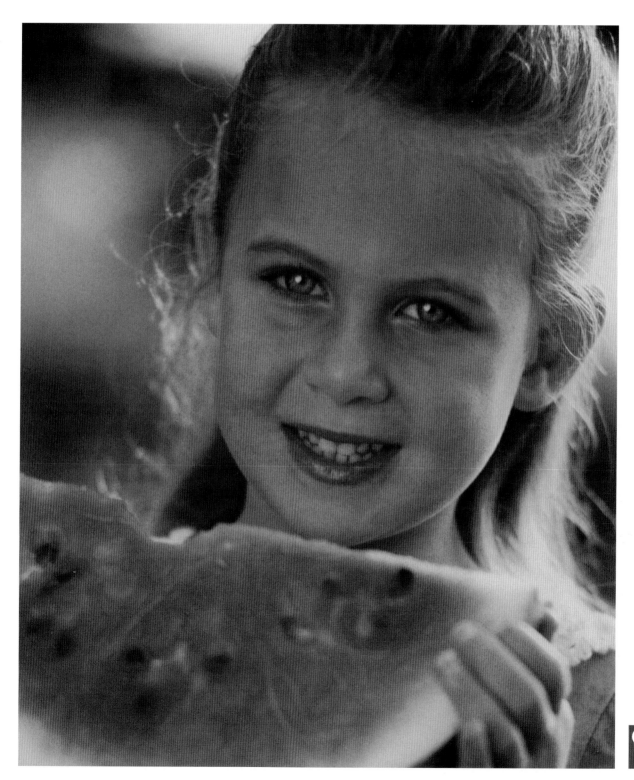

Earaches

An earache – technically known as **otitis media** (middle ear infection) – is *the* most common medical problem among young children today, accounting for more than 50% of all visits to pediatricians. The acute form (usually preceded by upper respiratory infection or allergy) will affect 66% of American children by age two, while the chronic form (constant swelling in the middle ear) will affect an equal number by age six.[1]

Although the standard of medical care for the condition involves use of antibiotics, analgesics (pain medication) and/or antihistamines and sometimes surgery (**myringotomy** – tubes in the ears – to drain fluid into the throat), numerous studies have shown that these methods were no more successful than a **placebo** (inactive substance) in alleviating symptoms.[2] These treatments, of course, are addressing the symptoms and not the cause and, in many instances, creating conditions for development of more serious problems.

To treat the cause, it must first be identified. As in so many other disorders, food allergies appear to have a direct relationship to ear infections. In fact, "most studies show that 85% to 93% of children with chronic otitis media have allergies – 16% to inhalants, 14% to food and 70% to both."[3] Previous chapters have noted the relationship of food allergies and sensitivities to poor digestion – how undigested proteins entering the circulation trigger an autoimmune allergic response.

Natural therapies, aimed at boosting immunity by treating food allergies, have a much better track record than drugs and surgery for treating ear infections, with "elimination of food allergens resulting in a dramatic effect in over 90% of children in some studies."[4] The same natural means of

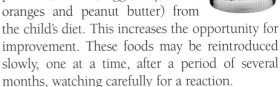

diagnosing and treating food and environmental allergies and sensitivities used in adults may be used for children – i.e., ELISA blood test, elimination diet and food rotation (so that no one food family is eaten too often), desensitization techniques (such as allergy shots). In the absence of testing, one may simply remove the most common allergens (milk and dairy products, wheat, eggs, soy, corn, oranges and peanut butter) from

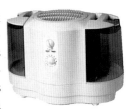

the child's diet. This increases the opportunity for improvement. These foods may be reintroduced slowly, one at a time, after a period of several months, watching carefully for a reaction.

Chances of improvement are especially good if additional supportive measures are taken: Add fresh vegetable juices to the child's diet (see chapter 8), use a humidifier if the air is dry, eliminate sugar from the child's diet (it's immunosuppressive); instead of sugar, use the South American herb stevia or the Chinese herb lo han. Additionally, supplements like thymus extract (500 mg. per day), liquid zinc sulfate (1–2 mg. four times a day) and vitamin C with bioflavonoids (50 mg. every two hours while symptoms are severe) can help enhance the immune system.

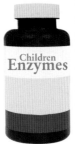

Children Enzymes

Since impaired digestion is a root cause of food allergies, it is also very important to help the child's digestion with a good plant-based enzyme taken with meals. Additionally, use of a probiotic to supplement the child's intestinal flora is recommended; this is especially important if antibiotics have been used.

be treated with chelation, a process whereby a substance is used either orally or intravenously to attract the metal and bind to it so it can be eliminated from the body. There are adult oral chelation products on the market that are natural blends of herbs, vitamins, minerals and amino acids designed to support a healthy mineral balance in the body. Though the formulas are designed for adults, they can be often used safely with children by just reducing the dose based on the child's weight: i.e., if the child weighs 75 pounds, and the product is based on a 150-pound person, a half dose would be given.

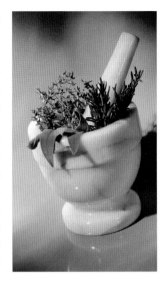

Heavy metals are abundant in the environment. Often they're found in the places we would least suspect, like childhood vaccines.

Vaccinations

There has been much controversy recently regarding the use of thimerosal-containing vaccines on children because of the mercury content (nearly 50%) of this preservative. **Thimerosal** is commonly used in vaccines to prevent them from spoiling; it also inactivates the bacteria that are used to formulate several vaccines and prevents bacterial contamination of the vaccine. The controversy about thimerosal reached a climax in the summer of 1999, when the American Academy of Pediatrics issued a joint statement in conjunction with the U.S. Public Health Service. It alerted physicians and the general public to the possible health threat posed by the presence of ethyl mercury (as thimerosal) in some vaccines recommended routinely for children in the U.S.

The EPA (Environmental Protection Agency) has established 'safe' levels of mercury as .1 microgram per 1.0 kilogram of body weight per day. Vaccines contain 12.5 to 25.0 micrograms of mercury. Therefore, during the course of a 'well baby' office visit, a child could have between 50–62.5 mcgs. of mercury injected directly into his or her bloodstream.[12]

There is a suspected link between autism (a neurological disorder characterized by impaired cognitive, social and language development) and thimerosal. Symptoms of mercury toxicity in young children are quite similar to those of autism. The increase in the number of children diagnosed as autistic seems to correlate with the introduction of hepatitis B and HIB (Haemophilus influenza, type B) vaccination of infants in the early 1990s.

Vaccinations are not the only source of mercury. It is commonly found in dental amalgam used to fill cavities in teeth. Vapors from the mercury used in dental fillings are decidedly toxic. These vapors, inhaled by a pregnant woman, can cause brain damage to the developing fetus, which can later manifest as learning disability, autism and/or ADD/ADHD. The infant who is exposed to mercury in utero via the mother's 'silver' filling vapors (which are emitted every time she chews), and is then given a thimerosal-containing vaccination soon after birth, is exposed to an extraordinary amount of toxicity.

The dangers from vaccinations are not limited to the damage done by thimerosal, however. In addition to mercury, vaccines typically contain a live or killed infectious agent (usually a virus or bacteria), other preservatives (notably formaldehyde), stabilizers, antibiotics and adjuvants (such as aluminum phosphate – another toxic metal!). Hannah Allen stated that the materials from which 'vaccines, serums and biologicals' are produced include such toxic components as diseased foreign tissue.[13]

There are many fine books on the market and sites on the World Wide Web with information on the dangers of immunizations and how to legally avoid them. We recommended *Immunization Theory and Reality* by Neil Z. Miller and *The Vaccine Guide: Making an Informed Choice* by Randall Neustaedter, and http://thinktwice.com/global.htm and www.garynull.com/market place/documents.asp on the web.

Food Additives

The late pediatric allergist, Dr. Benjamin Feingold, was one of the first healthcare professionals to recognize a connection between food additives and ADD. In 1973, he reported to an AMA gathering that more than half of his hyperactive patients had improved on a diet devoid of artificial flavors and colors and chemical preservatives. Ironically, both Ritalin and Cylert, two commonly prescribed medications for ADHD, contain artificial color! Dr. Feingold found that many hyperactive children react to chemical compounds (salicylates and phenolics, which occur naturally in foods) and improve when foods containing these are avoided.

The U.S. uses approximately 5,000 additives in food – that's about 8–10 pounds per person per year.[14] Many of the studies that examine the effects of these additives have been funded by major food manufacturers in this country (who use them in their products). This being the case, it's understandable

that Dr. Feingold's findings regarding food additives have not been consistently supported in controlled U.S. studies. It is noteworthy, however, that studies outside the U.S. *do* support the efficacy of his diet, and, most significantly, many hyperactive children have improved by following it. More information on the Feingold diet is available from the Feingold Association of the U.S. at 631-369-9340 (www.feingold.org).

While Dr. Feingold has provided a big piece of the ADHD puzzle, a shortcoming of his diet is that it fails to address the issues of food allergy and nutrient deficiency.

Food Allergies

Studies of food allergies and sensitivities in hyperactive children have shown that artificial food colors and preservatives are among the most reactive of food substances. Eliminating them from the diet may be helpful, but frequently there are other reactive foods that must be eliminated as well. The major ones are cow's milk, soy products, chocolate, oranges, grapes, peanuts, wheat, corn, tomatoes and cane sugar.

Pediatrician, Doris Rapp, in her book *The Impossible Child*, and in the accompanying video (available through Practical Allergy Research Foundation, 1-800-787-8780), shows dramatically how hyperactivity (and other conditions) starts and stops. She uses a **provocation/neutralization** technique, wherein a small amount of the reactive food (or chemical) is introduced sublingually (under the tongue). One concentration of the allergen will trigger the maladaptive response, while another will eliminate it. In D. Rapp's video, children can be seen behaving normally until an allergen is introduced. Immediately, they exhibit classic ADHD behaviors and even show signs of learning disabilities. The child who wrote normally before ingesting the allergen, inverted letters afterwards. Dr. Rapp also notes that children with such food sensitivities often have distinctive physical signs: circles, bags or wrinkles under the eyes and/or a horizontal crease across the bridge of the nose.

Refined Sugar

Sugar is one of the common allergens in hyperactive children. Even in the absence of an actual allergy or sensitivity, too much sucrose causes unstable blood sugar levels, which can affect the mood and behavior. One study found abnormal glucose tolerance curves, predominantly hypoglycemia (low blood sugar), in 74% of 261 hyperactive children.[15] Because hypoglycemia increases adrenaline secretion, it can contribute to hyperactivity. It can, of course, also lead to an overgrowth of Candida albicans. Where Candida is a problem, sugar and other sweeteners must be temporarily eliminated from the diet. In the absence of Candida, sweetening children's food with the herb lo han is recommended. It does not have the adverse effects of other sweeteners and actually helps to stabilize blood sugar levels. The same may be said of stevia, another good herbal alternative.

Candida and Parasites

As noted, Candida overgrowth is frequently the result of antibiotic overuse. Because the allergy and sugar components are so strong in ADD, the development of systemic candidiasis is not a surprising result. Recent studies and a wealth of clinical data show a close relationship between Candida overgrowth and ADD or ADHD. The diagnosis of ADD or ADHD is a red flag that Candida overgrowth and/or parasites may be a problem. Other red flags include:

- Thrush (oral Candida)
- Colic
- Recurring ear infections
- Chronic cough
- Headache
- Constipation
- Gas & bloating
- Mood swings
- Fatigue
- Allergies
- Diaper rash
- Irritability
- Nasal congestion
- Wheezing
- Digestive problems
- Diarrhea
- Craving for sweets
- Rectal itching
- Coated tongue
- Skin problems

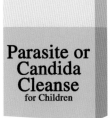

Dr. William Crook, well known for his book *The Yeast Connection*, has observed the presence of fungal metabolites in the urine of ADD and ADHD children. Typically, these children have a history of multiple antibiotic use. They have been helped, Dr. Crook has found, by a sugar-free diet and anti-fungal medication. The same diet used for adults may be used with children. The questionnaire in the appendix of this book will help assess a child's Candida risk. (Note: The adult questionnaire should not be confused with the one for children.)

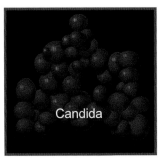

Candida

While anti-fungal medications can help control the Candida problem, it is always at a cost, because all drugs have undesirable side effects. A safer approach in treating children for Candida is the use of an herbal formula. Since, as previously observed, parasites most commonly accompany Candida, one would do well to

12

address both at the same time. It is particularly important with children to treat for parasites, as children are more susceptible to them than adults for a number of reasons:

- Children have a tendency to put their hands in their mouths much more frequently than adults. The parasites on hands and under fingernails are then transported directly into the system. Playing with animals and putting hands to the mouth can be a problem.

- Children's stomachs tend to be low in HCl, which is needed to help eliminate parasites when they enter the system.

- Many children have had multiple rounds of antibiotics, which create bacterial imbalance in the digestive tract, a state ideal for parasites.

- Day care centers in America are rife with parasitic infection. The Center for Disease Control states that some areas of the country report as many as 50% of day care children to be infected. Parasites can be spread during diaper changing and from child to child. Additional reports state that approximately 20% of parents become infected with parasites themselves while caring for sick children.

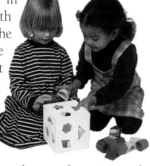

Candida overgrowth and parasites are serious health risks for children. Clinical reports suggest that a weakened immune system and a toxic bloodstream may cause widespread systemic and nervous system disturbances. These can lead to many problems, not the least of which is a repeat of ear infections and flu-like symptoms. If these conditions are treated with antibiotics, the situation is made worse, and the child experiences a spiraling cycle of decline.

If your child suffers from frequent colds, flu, ear infections, or allergies, has been labeled ADHD or shows other signs of parasites or Candida, here are some steps you can take now:

- Change the child's diet. Eliminate dairy products, sugar, wheat, corn and any products that contain preservatives or food colorings. Some good substitutes are millet, spelt, rice and quinoa. Ezekiel bread is also a tasty substitute for wheat breads.

- Vegetables are important as healing and rebuilding foods. Vegetables should be cleaned well with a vegetable wash (available from the health food store) or with diluted hydrogen peroxide.

- Start the child on a cleansing program to kill the Candida and parasites from which (s)he may be suffering. A special children's formula will help to remove these pathogens. A good formula would include such ingredients as **black walnut** (aids digestion, cleanses the body of parasites), **quassia** (used in the expulsion of threadworms and stimulates production of digestive juices), **garlic** (an anti-fungal), **cloves** (has antiseptic and anti-parasitic properties), **pippli** (used in India as an anti-parasitic), **wormwood** (expels worms), **pumpkin seed** (anti-parasitic) and **thyme** (anti-fungal and anti-parasitic).

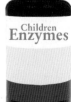

- Supplement the child's digestive process with a good **plant-based**

enzyme formula, one which includes amylase, lipase, protease and cellulase and may also include **papain** (from papaya), **bromelain** (from pineapple) and **pepsin** (breaks down protein) to aid digestion, as well as **L-glutamine** and **N-acetyl-glucosamine (NAG)** and **butyric acid** to help regenerate the intestinal lining.

- Supplement the child's intestinal flora with a good chewable probiotic formula that includes resident strains of beneficial bacteria that will implant in the intestines. These would include **Lactobacillus acidophilus, Bifidobacterium bifidum** and **Bifidobacterium infantis.** A prebiotic, such as **FOS,** will help feed these flora, while added **L-glutamine** and **NAG** will help restore the integrity of the intestinal mucosa.

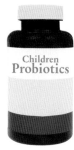

- If your child is not eliminating regularly (at least once a day), it is highly recommended that you take measures to normalize elimination naturally. A children's herbal laxative formula, containing such food concentrates as **flax seed, prune fruit, fig fruit, rhubarb root** and **peach leaf** will help in this regard. Herbs such as cascara sagrada or senna, which can over-stimulate the bowel, should be avoided.

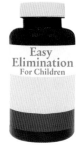

Getting a child successfully through a cleansing program may require considerable patience and persistence on the part of both the child and the parents. From my experience, it is easiest to stick to a program like this when the whole family is participating. The child is much more likely to cooperate when (s)he can see the whole family is doing it. Besides – there is a strong likelihood that if a child has Candida or parasites, the parents do too!

Fluorescent Lights

In the 1970s, John Ott did some pioneering research on the effects of light and other radiation on human health and behavior. His work began with plants, then animals, and moved finally to humans. In 1973, he found that when he exposed rats to the radiation from color TV sets, they became "increasingly hyperactive and aggressive within three to ten days, then progressively lethargic. By 30 days, they were so lethargic, they had to be pushed to move around the cage."[16] Such response is reminiscent of the child who is hypnotically glued to the TV set regardless of program content.

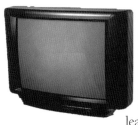

According to Ott, the same kind of radiation that comes from color TV sets also escapes from the cathodes of fluorescent lights. He also found that lead stopped these emissions of radiation. Another problem with fluorescents is that they contain an imbalance of the wavelengths that emit 'white' light. Ott helped establish the fact that the human body needs exposure to **full-pectrum light** (like sunlight), which is naturally balanced in its wavelength composition.

Dr. Ott instituted lighting experiments in classrooms in a Sarasota, Florida school in the 1970s to prove his point. Two windowless classrooms were outfitted with full-spectrum lights, while two others used conventional cool white fluorescent lights. Hidden time-lapse video cameras were used to observe the children's behavior in both classrooms during a period of five months. The behavior of the children exposed to the full-spectrum lights improved significantly, as did their general attendance, learning ability and concentration,[17] while no such improvement was noted in the children exposed to fluorescent lights. Further studies have confirmed these results, and full-spectrum lights are now being used in many progressive institutions.

In view of John Ott's findings, light and radiation may be considered added stress factors that contribute to ADD/ADHD in children.

Craniosacral Dysfunction

The 'craniosacral' system includes the brain and spinal cord (as well as the membranes surrounding them), cerebrospinal fluid and the bones of the skull and spine. Pioneering work in this field has been done by Dr. John Upledger who reports successfully treating hyperactive children with craniosacral therapy, a system of gentle manipulation of the cranial bones to restore them to their proper positioning. He states that in his experience more than half of ADD/ADHD behavior has its roots in the craniosacral system. His institute (Upledger Institute, 561-622-4334; www.upledger.com) offers intensive programs for children with ADD and learning disabilities.

Another approach to addressing craniosacral dysfunction is a specialized cranial manipulation technique called 'NeuroCranial Restructuring,' developed as a refinement of an old osteopathic technique (Bilateral Nasal Specific) by Dr. Dean Howell. NCR treatment results in a widening of the skull, an improvement in the flow of cerebrospinal fluid, and thus an improvement in brain activity, according to Dr. Howell who claims that NCR creates bone changes that cannot be accomplished with craniosacral therapy. *Dynamic Healing through NeuroCranial Restructuring* (Power of One Publishing, 1-800-830-4778, ext. 246) has more information on this technique.

Notes

[1] Michael Murray, ND, *Encyclopedia of Natural Medicine*, Prina Publishing, 1998, p. 440.

[2] Ibid., p. 442.

[3] Ibid., p. 443-444.

[4] Ibid., p. 443.

[5] Ibid.

[6] Ibid., p. 442.

[7] Ibid., p. 273.

[8] Susan Stockton, *ADD: It Doesn't Add Up*, Power of One Publishing, 1997, p. 9.

[9] Ibid., p. 7.

[10] Ibid., p. 8.

[11] Op. Cit., Murray, p. 278-279.

[12] Alan Yurko, 'Vaccines – Injection of Death,' *Crusader*, Feb.- Mar., 2002, p. 12-16.

[13] Hannah Allen, *Don't Get Stuck*, Hygiene Press, 1985, p. 222.

[14] Ibid., p. 274.

[15] Ibid., p. 277.

[16] John Ott, *Health and Light*, Pocket Books, 1973, p. 127.

[17] Ibid., p. 192.

Chapter Summary

This chapter has presented information on how common childhood disorders – earache and ADD/ ADHD – can have their roots in GI dysfunction related to impaired digestion. Some of the underlying causes of these disorders – disruption of intestinal flora, food allergies, systemic candidiasis, parasites – are the same as the underlying causes in more serious 'adult' diseases, like IBS, discussed in chapter 11.

Standard medical treatment of ear infection (antibiotics) and ADD/ADHD (Ritalin) not only fails to correct the cause of these disorders, but it also can exacerbate the conditions and/or compromise the overall health of the child with serious side effects. Conversely, safe natural approaches to healing and restoration of balance – high fiber, non-allergenic foods, enzyme and probiotic supplements and herbal detox formulas – can be used successfully with children of all ages.

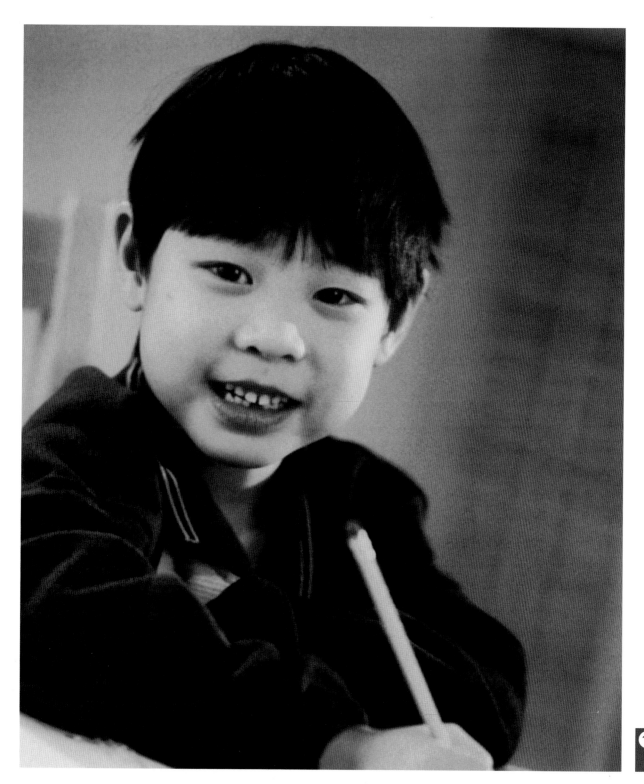

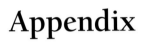

Appendix

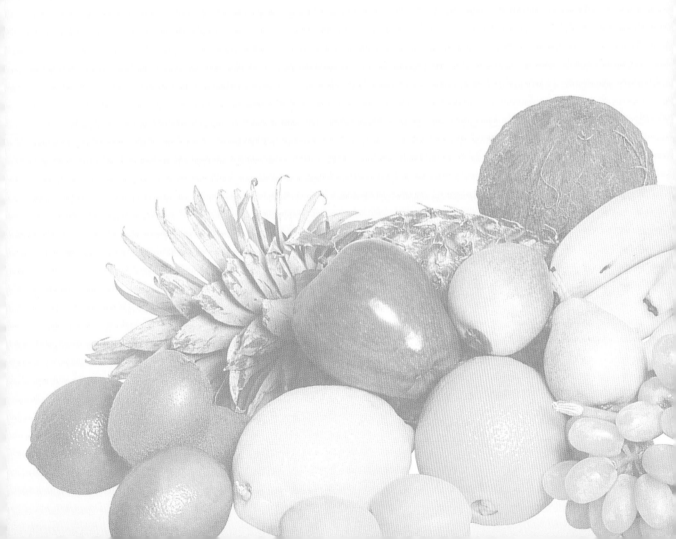

Yeast Questionnaire – Adult

Section A – History

Circle the number next to the questions you answer 'yes,' then add all the circled numbers and write the total in the box at the bottom.

1. Have you taken tetracycline (Sumycin®, Panmycin®, Vibramycin®, Minocin®, etc.) or other antibiotics for acne for 1 month or more? 50

2. Have you at any time in your life, taken other "broad spectrum" antibiotics for respiratory, urinary or other infections for 2 months or more, or for shorter periods, 4 or more times in a 1-year span? . . .50

3. Have you taken a broad spectrum antibiotic drug – even for 1 period? 6

4. Have you at any time in your life, been bothered by persistent prostatitis, vaginitis, or other problems affecting your reproductive organs? 25

5. Have you been pregnant...
   a) 2 or more times? 5
   b) 1 time? 3

6. Have you taken birth control pills for...
   a) more than 2 years? 15
   b) 6 months to 2 years? .8

7. Have you taken prednisone, Decadron® or other cortisone-type drugs by mouth or inhalation...
   a) for more than 2 weeks? 15
   b) for 2 weeks or less? 6

8. Does exposure to perfumes, insecticides, fabric shop odors, or other chemicals provoke...
   a) moderate to severe symptoms? 20
   b) mild symptoms? 5

9. Are your symptoms worse on damp, muggy days or in moldy places? 20

10. If you have ever had athlete's foot, ringworm, jock itch or other chronic fungus infections of the skin or nails, have such infections been...
    a) severe or persistent? .20
    b) mild or moderate? 10

11. Do you crave sugar? 10

12. Do you crave breads? 10

13. Do you crave alcoholic beverages? 10

14. Does tobacco smoke really bother you? 10

Section B – Major Symptoms

For each symptom that is present, enter the appropriate number on the adjacent line:

- If a symptom is occasional or mild, **score 3 points**
- If a symptom is frequent or moderately severe, **score 6 points**
- If a symptom is severe and/or disabling, **score 9 points**

Total the scores for this section and record them in the box at the bottom of this section.

1. Fatigue or lethargy . . . . .____
2. Feeling of being 'drained' . . . . .____
3. Poor memory . . . . .____
4. Feeling 'spacey' or 'unreal' . . . . .____
5. Inability to make decisions . . . . .____
6. Numbness, burning or tingling . . . . .____
7. Insomnia . . . . .____
8. Muscle aches . . . . .____
9. Muscle weakness or paralysis . . . . .____
10. Pain and/or swelling in joints . . . . .____
11. Abdominal pain . . . . .____
12. Constipation . . . . .____
13. Diarrhea . . . . .____
14. Bloating, belching or intestinal gas . . . . .____
15. Troublesome vaginal burning, itching or discharge .____
16. Prostatitis . . . . .____
17. Impotence . . . . .____
18. Loss of sexual desire or feeling . . . . .____
19. Endometriosis or infertility . . . . .____
20. Cramps and/or other menstrual irregularities . . . . .____
21. Premenstrual tension .____
22. Attacks of anxiety or crying . . . . .____
23. Cold hands or feet and/or chilliness . . . . .____
23. Shaking or irritability when hungry . . . . .____

Total Score for Section A: _____

Total Score for Section B: _____

Section C – Minor Symptoms

For each symptom that is present, enter the appropriate number on the adjacent line:

- If a symptom is occasional or mild,
  score 3 points
- If a symptom is frequent or moderately severe,
  score 6 points
- If a symptom is severe and/or disabling,
  score 9 points

Total the scores for this section and record them in the box at the bottom of this section.

1. Drowsy . . . . .____
2. Irritable or jittery .____
3. Lack of coordination . . . . .____
4. Inability to concentrate . . . . .____
5. Frequent mood swings . . . . .____
6. Headaches . . . . .____
7. Dizzy/loss of balance . . . . .____
8. Pressure above ears...feeling of head swelling . . . .____
9. Tendency to bruise easily . . . . .____
10. Chronic rashes or itching . . . . .____
11. Psoriasis or recurrent hives . . . . .____
12. Indigestion or heartburn . . . . .____
13. Food sensitivity or intolerance . . . . .____
14. Mucus in stools . . . . .____
15. Rectal itching . . . . .____
16. Dry mouth or throat . . . . .____
17. Rash or blisters in mouth . . . . .____
18. Bad breath . . . . .____
19. Foot, hair or body odor not relieved by washing . .____
20. Nasal congestion or post-nasal drip . . . . .____
21. Nasal itching . . . . .____
22. Sore throat . . . . .____
23. Laryngitis, loss of voice . . . . .____
24. Cough or recurrent bronchitis . . . . .____
25. Pain or tightness in chest . . . . .____
26. Wheezing or shortness of breath . . . . .____
27. Urinary frequency, urgency or incontinence . . . . .____
28. Burning on urination . . . . .____
29. Spots in front of eyes or erratic vision . . . . .____
30. Burning or tearing of eyes . . . . .____
31. Recurrent infections or fluid in ears . . . . .____
32. Ear pain or deafness . . . . .____

Total Score for Section C: _____

GRAND TOTAL SCORE: _____

IF YOUR SCORE IS:	YOUR SYMPTOMS ARE:
180 (women) 140 (men)	Almost certainly yeast connected
120 (women) 90 (men)	Probably yeast connected
60 (women) 40 (men)	Possibly yeast connected
below 60 (women) below 40 (men)	Probably not yeast connected

The total score will help you and your physician decide if your health problems are yeast-connected. A comprehensive history and physical examination are also important. In addition, laboratory studies, x-rays, and other types of tests may also be appropriate.

Scores for women will be higher, as 7 items in this questionnaire apply exclusively to women, while only 2 apply exclusively to men.

If your total score for all three sections above was less than 60 for a woman or less than 40 for a man, then you are less likely to have a problem with Candida. However, if you scored higher than this then you may wish to consider lifestyle and dietary changes, as well as a detoxification and cleansing program, all of which may help you feel healthy and more energetic.

Reprinted from *The Yeast Connection* by William G. Crook, MD with permission.

Yeast Questionnaire – Child

Circle appropriate point score for questions you answer "yes." Total your score and record it at the end of the questionnaire.

Point Score

1.   During the two years before your child was born, were you bothered by recurrent vaginitis, menstrual irregularities, premenstrual tension, fatigue, headache, depression, digestive disorders of 'feeling bad all over?' 30

2.   Was your child bothered by thrush? (Score 10 if mild, score 20 if severe or persistent) 10/20

3.   Was your child bothered by frequent diaper rashes in infancy? (Score 10 if mild, 20 if severe or persistent) 10/20

4.   During infancy, was your child bothered by colic and irritability lasting over 3 months? (Score 10 if mild, 20 if moderate or severe) 10/20

5.   Are his/her symptoms worse on damp days or in damp or moldy places? 20

6.   Has your child been bothered by recurrent or persistent 'athlete's foot' or chronic fungus infections of his skin or nails? 30

7.   Has your child been bothered by recurrent hives, eczema or other skin problems? 10

8.   Has your child received:

   (a) 4 or more courses of antibiotic drugs during the past year? Or has he received continuous 'prophylactic' courses of antibiotic drugs? 80

   (b) 8 or more courses of 'broad-spectrum' antibiotics (such as amoxicillin, Keflex®, Septra®, Bactrim® or Ceclor®) during the past 3 years? 50

9.   Has your child experienced recurrent ear problems? 10

10. Has your child had tubes inserted in his ears? 10

11. Has your child been labeled 'hyperactive?' (Score 10 if mild, 20 if moderate or severe) 10/20

12. Is your child bothered by learning problems (even though his early developmental history was normal)? 10

13. Does your child have a short attention span? 10

14. Is your child persistently irritable, unhappy and hard to please? 10

15. Has your child been bothered by persistent or recurrent digestive problems, including constipation, diarrhea, bloating or excessive gas? (Score 10 if mild, 20 if moderate, 30 if severe) 10/20/30

16.   Has he/she been bothered by persistent nasal congestion, cough and/or wheezing? 10

17.   Is your child unusually tired or unhappy or depressed? (Score 10 if mild, 20 if servere) 10/20

18.   Has your child been bothered by recurrent headaches, abdominal pain or muscle aches?
      (Score 10 if mild, 20 if severe) 10/20

19.   Does your child crave sweets? 10

20.   Does exposure to perfume, insecticides, gas or other chemicals provoke moderate to
      severe symptoms? 30

21.   Does tobacco smoke really bother him? 20

22.   Do you feel that your child isn't well, yet diagnostic tests and studies haven't revealed the cause? 10

TOTAL SCORE: _____

Yeasts possibly play a role in causing health problems in children with
scores of 60 or more.

Yeasts probably play a role in causing health problems in children with
scores of 100 or more.

Yeasts almost certainly play a role in causing health problems in children with
scores of 140 or more.

Cultured Vegetable Recipe

Taken from *The Body Ecology Diet* by Donna Gates

Step 1 – Use mostly cabbage (organic, green and/or red), either by itself or with beets, carrots, garlic, celery, red peppers, kelp, herbs (thyme, dill), or any other vegetable you want. Use a minimum of 10 heads of cabbage.

Grind them up with a food processor. Then place them into a large stainless steel bowl and pound them with a bat or a similar heavy, blunt object until they become a little juicy. While beating, add freshly squeezed lemon juice. (See recipe on next page).

A Champion® juicer works well for grinding vegetables, but be sure to grind them with the blank plastic piece and not the screen. This blank piece lets you grind without juicing. If you use the Champion juicer you will not need to pound the cabbage with a bat.

Step 2 – Put the vegetables into a stainless steel, ceramic, or glass crock. Don't fill the crock to the brim, because the fermenting vegetables are likely to expand and overflow.

Step 3 – Put a large portion of fresh cabbage leaves on top of the ground-up vegetables (completely covering the ground-up vegetables).

Step 4 – With your hands and a little body weight, gently, yet firmly and evenly, compress the leaves.

Step 5 – Put a plate that is as wide as possible in the crock.

Step 6 – Put some weight on the plate. You can use a jar or something else that has some weight to it. We like to use a jar that won't leak, filled with about two-thirds of a pint of water. A little weight is good but don't put on so much that vegetable juice is forced up above the fermenting vegetables. You want to check the fermenting vegetables a few times in the next 24-36 hours to confirm you have the right amount of weight and to make sure that the plate is sitting on the vegetables evenly.

Step 7 – Cover the crock with a clean dish towel. Let the fermenting vegetables sit in a well-ventilated room at room temperature (between 60-70 degrees) for five to seven days. The longer they sit, the stronger they become. After five to seven days (6-7 days at 60 degrees and 5-6 days at 70 degrees), throw away the old cabbage leaves and moldy and discolored vegetables on the top. Put the remaining fermented vegetables in glass jars and refrigerate. This raw sauerkraut will last from four to eight months when kept at 34 degrees and opened minimally. Do not freeze.

A Beginner's Recipe
Taken from *The Body Ecology Diet* by Donna Gates

We like to add freshly squeezed lemon juice to our cabbage because it tastes delicious and retains the beautiful color in the vegetables. Here is our favorite beginner's recipe:

For every three heads of cabbage: (We use two green cabbages and one red cabbage)

Combine 3/4 to 1 cup freshly squeezed lemon juice and 3 tablespoons dried dill weed.

Put this mixture into a stainless steel bowl, and beat it thoroughly with a blunt object. Put this into a crock or stainless steel stockpot, and cover with at least two layers of cabbage leaves, the plate and the heavy object. Find a cool spot in your house, and let it sit for six days before unveiling it. Scrape off any foam or mildew from the top or edges, and refrigerate as above. Your batch, if you've made it correctly, should be brightly colored, juicy and sweet.

If you want to add other vegetables, use a layering method:

Grate vegetables in a food processor. Add more lemon juice and more dill (or other herbs), and then pound them as explained above. Layer cabbage in the bottom of a large pot or crock about six inches deep, then add layers of carrots, peppers, beets, celery, daikon, onions, then a layer of cabbage, etc.

Press down each layer so the vegetables will be saturated in their own juice. When the container is full, cover it with the cabbage leaves, a plate, a heavy stone or weight and a dishcloth, and continue as above.

If you want to make another batch right away, some connoisseurs recommend starting your next batch of raw cultured vegetables in the same empty pot or crock without washing it each time.

You will improve your technique with each batch you make.

Resource Directory

ADD/ADHD

Feingold® Association of the United States
631-369-9340
www.feingold.org

Dr. Doris Rapp
Practical Allergy Research Foundation
P.O. Box 60
Buffalo, NY 14223

Books

ADDiction & Attention Deficit Disorder – Susan Stockton, Power of One Publishing (1-800-830-4778, ext. 246)

Beyond Amalgam: The Health Hazard Posed by Jawbone Cavitations – Susan Stockton, Power of One Publishing (1-800-830-4778, ext. 246)

Candida Made Simple – Cheryl Townsley, LFH Publishing (303-794-1449)

Conquer Candida – Jack Tips, ND, Ph.D., Apple-A-Day Press (512-328-3996)

Digestive Wellness – Elizabeth Lipski, MS, CCN, Keats Publishing

Dynamic Healing through NeuroCranial Restructuring – Susan Stockton, Power of One Publishing (1-800-4778, ext. 246)

Immunization Theory & Reality – Neil Z. Miller, Thinktwice Global Vaccine Institute (505-983-1856)

Juicing for Life – Cherie Calbhom & Maureen Keane, Avery Publishing

Nourishing Traditions – Sally Fallon, ProMotion Publishing (1-800-231-1776)

Root Canal Cover-Up – George Meinig, DDS (available thru PPNF, 1-800-366-3748)

The Candida Albicans Yeast-Free Cookbook – Pat Connolly, PPNF (1-800-366-3748)

The Body Ecology Diet – Donna Gates, B.E.D. Publications (1-800-511-2660)

The Impossible Child – Dr. Doris Rapp, Practical Allergy Research (1-800-787-8780)

The Mysterious Cause of Illness – John Matsen, ND, Fischer Publishing

The Pro Vita! Plan – Jack Tips, ND, PhD, Apple-A-Day Press (512-328-3996)

The Terrain is Everything – Susan Stockton, Power of One Publishing (1-800-830-4778, Ext. 246)

The Yeast Connection – Dr. William Crook (IHF – 660-7090)

Your Body's Many Cries for Water – F. Batmanghelidj, MD, Global Health Solutions

Candida Information
http://candida-yeast.com

Castor Oil Pack Kit
The Heritage Store
P.O. Box 444
Virginia Beach, VA 23458-0444
1-800-862-2923
www.caycecures.com

Charcoal
New Lifestyle Health Products
30 Uchee Pines Rd, Ste. 15
Seale, AL 36875
1-800-542-5695

Clay (for Detox Baths)
LL's Magnetic Clay
1-800-257-3315
www.magneticclay.com

Chemical Sensitivities
Dr. Gloria Gilbère
Naturopathic Health and Research Center
P.O. Box 3220
7098 Ash St.
Bonners Ferry, ID 83805
208-267-5417
www.drgloriagilbere.com

Colon Hydrotherapy
I-ACT
P.O. Box 461285
San Antonio, TX 78246-1285
210-366-2888
www.i-act.org

Colon Hydrotherapy Manufacturers (Closed Systems)
Clearwater Colon Hydrotherapy
4451-A South Pine Ave.
Ocala, FL 34480
352-401-0303
1-888-869-6191

Dotolo Research
2875 MCI Drive
Pinellas Park, FL 33782-6105
1-800-237-8458

Prime Pacific International QPW Ltd.
P.O. Box 87076
North Vancouver, B.C., Canada V7L 4P6
1-800-223-9374

Specialty Health
21636 N. 14th Ave., Suite A1
Phoenix, AZ 85027
623-582-4950

TRANSCOM S.L.
Sangroniz, 6, Edificio Beaz
Pabellon 15
48150 Sondika (Vizcaya), Spain
001 (34-4) 4531033
001 (34-4) 4710116

Colon Hydrotherapy Manufacturers (Open Systems)
Colon Therapeutics, Inc.
2909 Main Ave.
Groves, TX 77619
409-963-0300

Tiller MIND BODY, Inc.
10911 West Ave.
San Antonio, TX 78213
210-308-8888
800-939-1110

Craniosacral Therapy
The Upledger Institute, Inc.®
11211 Prosperity Farms Rd., Ste. D-325
Palm Beach Gardens, FL 33410
561-622-4334
www.upledger.com

Dental Information (Holistic) and Referral
DAMS (Dental Amalgam Mercury Syndrome)
P.O. Box 7249
Minneapolis, MN 55407-0249
1-800-311-6265
www.dams.cc

Electrolytes
Health Equations
P.O. Box 323
Newfane, VT 05345
1-800-328-2818
www.healtheqs.com

Environmental Products
Healthy Home Center
2435 9th St. North
St. Petersburg, FL 33704
1-800-583-9523
www.healthyhome.com

Food Safety
Food and Water, Inc.
P.O. Box 543
Montpelier, VT 05601
fax 802-229-6751
1-800-EAT-SAFE
www.foodandwater.org

Green Drinks
Greens Plus®
Orange Peel Enterprises
2183 Ponce de Leon Circle
Vero Beach, FL 32960
1-800-643-1210
www.greensplus.com

Perfect Food™
Garden of Life
1449 Jupiter Park Drive, Ste. 16
Jupiter, FL 33458
1-800-622-8986
fax 561-575-5488
www.gardenoflifeusa.com

Sweet Wheat, Inc.
P.O. Box 187
Clearwater, FL 33757
1-888-227-9338
fax 727-462-5454
www.sweetwheat.com

Herbal Cleansing Products
Renew Life Formulas, Inc.
2076 Sunnydale Blvd.
Clearwater, FL 33765
1-800-830-4778
www.renewlife.com

Hemorrhoids
Pilex®
25675 Meadowview Ct.
Salinas, CA 93908-9396
831-484-7820
1-800-745-3995 (10-8 EST)
fax: 831-484-2203
www.varicose.com

Kefir
Helios Nutrition Limited
318 The Decotah Building
370 Selby Ave.
St. Paul, MN 55102
651-298-8565
fax 651-298-0602

Laboratory Testing
Doctor's Data™ (nutritional, gastrointestinal, immunology, environmental testing)
3755 Illinois Ave.
St. Charles, IL 60174-2420
1-800-323-2784
www.doctorsdata.com

Great Smokies Diagnostic Laboratory/Genovations™
(endocrinology, gastrointestinal, immunology,
nutritional, metabolic testing)
63 Zillicoa St.
Asheville, NC 28801
1-800-522-4762
fax 1-828-252-9303
www.gsdl.com

NeuroCranial Restructuring

NeuroCranial Restructuring
c/o NCR-01
P.O. Box 448
Tonasket, WA 98855-0448
1-888-252-0411
fax 425-458-4319
www.ndnd.com

Nutrition

Price-Pottenger Nutrition Foundation
7890 Broadway
Lemon Grove, CA 91945
1-800-366-3748
fax 619-433-3136
www.price-pottenger.org

The Weston A. Price Foundation
4200 Wisconsin Ave., N.W.
Washington, DC 20007
202-333-HEAL
www.westonaprice.org

Sauna (Infrared)

TheraSauna™
1021 State St.
Bettendorf, IA 52722
1-888-729-7727
www.therasauna.com

Vaccinations

Thinktwice Global Vaccine Institute
P.O. Box 9638
Santa Fe, NM 87504
505-983-1856
Http://thinktwice.com/global.htm

Vacuum Packaging Systems

Tilia, Inc.™
P.O. Box 194530
San Francisco, CA 94119-4530
1-877-804-5383
www.foodsaver.com

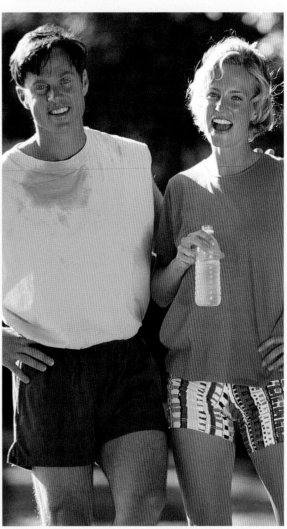

Bibliography

Batmanghelidj, F., MD. *Your Body's Many Cries for Water*. Global Health Solutions: Falls Church, VA, 1992.

Bieler, Henry F., MD. *Food is Your Best Medicine*. Ballantine Books: New York, 1965.

Bland, Jeffrey, Ph.D. *The 20-Day Rejuvenation Diet Program*. Keats Publishing, Inc.: New Canaan, Connecticut, 1997.

Braly, James, MD and Laura Torbet. *Dr. Braly's Food Allergy and Nutrition Revolution*. Keat's Publishing, Inc.: New Canaan, Connecticut, 1992.

Calbhom, Cherie and Maureen Keane, *Juicing for Life*. Avery, 1992.

Connolly, Pat. *The Candida Albicans Yeast-Free Cookbook*, 2nd Edition. Keats Publishing: Los Angeles, CA, 2000.

Erasmus, Udo. *Fats that Heal, Fats that Kill*. Alive Books: Burnaby BC Canada, 1993.

Fallon, Sally, *Nourishing Traditions*. Promotion Publishing: San Diego, CA, 1995.

Galland, Leo, MD. *The Four Pillars of Healing*. Random House: New York, 1997.

Gates, Donna. *The Body Ecology Diet*. B.E.D. Publications: Atlanta, GA, 1996.

Ghen, Mitchell J. *The Advanced Guide to Longevity Medicine*. Partners in Wellness: Landrum, SC, 2001.

Howell, Dr. Edward. *Enzyme Nutrition*. Avery Publishing Group, Inc.: Wayne, New Jersey, 1985.

Huggins, Hal, DDS, MS. *Detoxification*. Peak Energy Performance: Colorado Springs, CO.

Kaufmann, Doug A. *The Fungus Link*. MediaTrition: Rockwell, TX, 2000.

Kitchen, Judy, "Hypochlorhydria: A Review – Part I," *The Townsend Letter for Doctors and Patients*. October, 2001.

Kellas, William R., Ph.D and Andrea Sharon Dworkin, ND. *Surviving the Toxic Crisis*. Professional Preference: Olivenhain, CA, 1996.

Krohn, Jacqueline, MD and Frances Taylor, MA. *Natural Detoxification*. Hartley and Marks Publishers, Inc.: Vancouver, BC, Canada, 2000.

Lake, Rhody. *Liver Cleansing Handbook*. Alive Books: Vancouver, Canada, 2000.

Lipski, Elizabeth, MS, CCN. *Digestive Wellness*. Keats Publishing, Inc.: New Canaan, Connecticut, 1996.

Lorenzani, Shirley S., Ph.D. Candida: *A Twentieth Century Disease*. Keats Publishing: New Canaan, CT, 1986.

Matsen, Jonn, ND. *The Mysterious Cause of Illness*. Fischer Publishing Corporation: Canfield, Ohio, 1987.

Meinig, George E., DDS, FACD. *Root Canal Cover Up*. Bion Publishing: Ojai, CA, 1993.

Murray, Michael, ND and Joseph Pizzorno, ND. *Encyclopedia of Natural Medicine*. Prima Publishing, 1998.

Nichols, Trent W., MD and Nancy Faass, MSW, MPH, *Optimal Digestion*. Quill, An Imprint of Harper Collins Publishers, 2000.

Ott, John. *Health and Light*. Pocket Books: New York, New York, 1973.

Palmer, Melissa, MD. *Hepatitis and Liver Disease*. Avery Publishing Group: Garden City Park, New York, 2000.

Reams, Carey A. *Choose Life or Death*. Holistic Laboratories, Inc.: Tampa, FL., 1990.

Rockwell, Dr. Sally. *Coping with Candida Cookbook*. Sally J. Rockwell, Ph.D.: Seattle, Washington, 1996.

Stockton, Susan. *ADD: It Doesn't Add Up!* Power of One Publishing: Clearwater, FL, 1997.

Stockton, Susan. *Beyond Amalgam: The Health Hazard Posed by Jawbone Cavitations*, Third Printing. Power of One Publishing: Clearwater, FL, 2001.

Stockton, Susan. *Dynamic Healing through NeuroCranial Restructuring*. Power of One Publishing: Clearwater, FL, 1999.

Stockton, Susan. *The Terrain is Everything*. Power of One Publishing: Clearwater, FL, 2000.

Tips, Jack, ND, Ph.D. *Conquer Candida*. Apple-A-Day Press: Austin, TX, 1995.

Tips, Jack, ND, Ph.D. *The Pro Vita! Plan*. Apple-A-Day Press: Austin, TX, 1999.

Tips, Jack, ND, Ph.D. *Your Liver…Your Lifeline*. Apple-A-Day Press: Austin, TX, 1993.

Townsley, Cheryl. *Candida Made Simple*. LFH Publishing: Littleton, CO, 1999.

Townsley, Cheryl. *Cleansing Made Simple*. LFH Publishing: Littleton, CO, 2001 (revised edition).

Walker, Morton, DPM. "Value of Colon Hydrotherapy Verified by Medical Professionals Prescribing It." *Townsend Letter for Doctors and Patients*. August/September, 2000 (#205/206).

Webster, David. *Achieving Maximum Health*. Hygeia Publishing: Cardiff, CA, 1995.

Wilson, Denis, MS. *Doctor's Manual for Wilson's Syndrome*, 3rd Edition. Muskeegee Medical Publishing Company: USA, 1991.

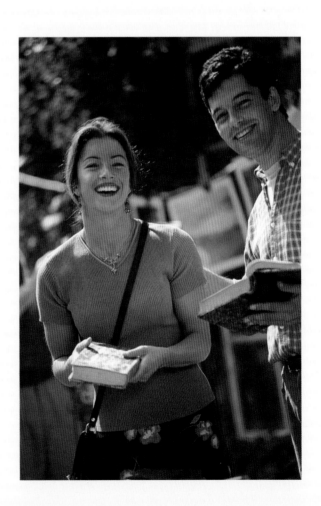

Index

Cigarette 15, 46, 49, 157
Cilantro leaf 117
Cleansing 14, 50, 53, 65, 67, 75, 77-81, 83, 84, 88-91, 93, 97-99,
     106-109, 111, 113, 116, 118, 119, 130, 133, 136, 142-
     144, 150-154, 163, 164
     Anti-fungal 97
Closed system 86
Cloves 99, 163
Cobalt 18, 46
Cocaine 45, 157
Coconut 126, 127, 134, 135
Coffee 55, 58, 77, 95, 135, 141, 147, 151
Cold-pressed 90, 113
Colds 163
Colitis 36, 39, 40, 75, 85, 139, 151-154
Colon 3, 8-10, 12-14, 24, 31, 37-39, 52, 55, 56, 59, 62-64, 75, 77,
     79-81, 83-86, 89, 90, 98, 100, 101, 109, 115, 116, 128, 140
     cancer 38, 69, 127, 140
Colonics 84
Commensal 37, 38
Congestion 143, 162
Conjugation 60, 63, 64
Constipation 22, 31, 36, 38-39, 41, 45, 46, 49, 50, 52, 56-57, 60,
     85, 125, 127, 129, 139-144, 146, 148, 150, 153-155,
     162
Conventional sauna 81, 82
Cooked Foods 121, 125, 126, 136
Copper 18, 60, 78, 159
Cortisone 33, 46, 93, 151
Cranberry fruit 147
Cranesbill 108, 110, 152
Crohn's disease 40, 139, 144
Cultured vegetables 95, 105
Cystine 131
Cytotoxic 46

D

Dairy products 20, 95, 96, 126, 128, 132, 134, 136, 145, 147, 152,
     158, 163
DAMS 48
Dandelion 79, 97, 114
Defecation 8
Deficiencies 20, 22, 24, 32, 39, 49, 51, 57, 105, 124, 148, 159
Degenerative disease 19, 36, 37, 64, 67, 119, 128
Deglycyrrhizinated licorice 73, 108, 150, 151
Dehydration 6, 56, 90, 125, 129, 142, 145
Delbrueckii 100
Deli meat 97
Dental amalgam mercury syndrome 48
Dentin tubules 47
Depression 32, 33, 117, 118, 124, 139, 140, 146, 157
Dermatitis 46, 106
Desensitization 158
Detox
     bath 83
     diet 70, 109
Detoxification 13, 33, 41, 43, 45, 4, 48, 52, 57-60, 62-65, 67, 75,
     77-79, 81, 82, 87-89, 111, 113, 116, 118, 119, 124,
     143, 150-152
DGL 73, 109, 150-152
Diabetes 36, 106, 127, 139, 146
Diaper rash 162

Diaphragm 13, 136
Diarrhea 22, 31, 36, 37, 41, 45, 46, 49, 80, 139, 144-148, 152,
     154, 162
Diet 15, 18, 23, 24, 27, 34, 38, 39, 63-65, 67, 70-73, 75, 77, 84,
     88, 91, 93, 94, 96-98, 105, 107-109, 111, 113, 114, 116, 118,
     119, 121, 125-136, 141, 142, 147, 150-154, 157, 158, 161-
     163
Dietary fiber 38, 41, 56, 101, 127, 128, 148
Digestion 3, 5-8, 10, 12, 14, 17-21, 24-27, 38, 49, 50, 53, 56, 63,
     65, 67-73, 81, 87, 93, 98, 102,103, 113, 119, 121, 128,
     134, 137, 139, 140, 146, 150, 152, 154, 158, 159, 163-
     164
Digestive
     diseases 140
     disorder 15, 26, 41, 126, 128
     enzyme 5-7, 14, 19, 24, 65, 67, 71, 73, 80, 98, 99, 119, 142,
          150, 153
     juices 27, 70, 136, 163
     organs 17, 18, 20, 21, 24, 26, 43, 48, 68, 71, 80, 125, 129
     stress 3, 17, 27, 31, 70, 73
     system 87, 89, 98, 102, 109, 113, 132, 140, 141
     toxins 55
Diuretics 45, 141
Diverticular disease 144, 146
Diverticulitis 85, 139, 153
Dosing the probiotic 102
Dry mouth 145
Duodenal ulcers 73, 139
Duodenum 6, 7, 14, 22-24, 57, 59, 151

E

Earache 155, 158, 165
Edema 46, 61
EFA 108, 154
Electrolyes 56
Electromagnetic pollution 48, 52
ELISA 146, 158
Emotional stress 17, 31, 38, 48, 155
Endorphins 69
Endotoxins 29, 39-41, 43, 53, 59, 60, 64
Enema 83, 84
Enteritis 41, 151
Environmental
     illness 51
     pollution 53, 61
     toxins 15, 27, 29, 31, 48, 52, 64, 67, 75, 119
Enzymes 5-7, 10, 14, 17, 20-24, 27, 46, 47, 50, 59, 60, 68-72, 78,
     87, 90, 101, 102, 105, 107, 109, 113-114, 120, 123, 125,
     133, 136, 145, 149, 150, 154
     supplementation 71
Esophagus 3, 5, 14, 73, 140, 149-151
Essential fatty acids 49, 80, 106, 124, 133, 141, 142
Exercise 69, 81, 84, 89
Ezekiel bread 90, 163

F

Faecalis 100
Faecium 100, 102
Feces 8, 115
Fever 61, 80, 145, 159
Fiber 8, 12, 18, 80, 81, 83, 87, 88, 98, 109, 111, 113, 118, 120,
     127-130, 136, 141, 142, 147, 148, 151-154, 165

Ileitis 151
Ileocecal valve 8, 14, 38
Ileum 7, 152
Imitation cheese 19
Immune system 25, 27, 31, 34, 36, 41, 53, 55, 58, 70, 71, 81, 89, 91, 93, 106, 117, 137, 139, 155, 158, 163
Impaired digestion 15, 17, 21, 31, 37, 39, 41, 43, 52, 55, 64, 121, 158, 165
Indigestion 18, 20, 21, 23, 25, 45, 53, 70, 72, 117, 139, 146, 149
Infantis 100, 104, 105, 164
Infertility 32, 33, 139
Inflammation 26, 27, 38-41, 46, 57, 61, 75, 97, 107-109, 143, 149, 151, 152, 154
Inflammatory bowel disease 9, 108, 144
Infrared sauna 81, 82
Insoluble fiber 80, 128, 129, 142
Insulin 7, 58, 101, 124
Interstitial cystitis 32
Intestinal
    disorders 32
    gas 9
    lining 26, 39, 46, 55, 98, 107, 109, 164
    mucosa 39, 41, 68, 77, 91, 93, 106, 107, 164
    permeability 25, 29, 32, 34, 45, 68, 129
    toxemia 17, 27, 29, 31, 37, 39, 41, 55, 150
    toxins 29, 41, 43, 61, 64
    tract 9, 10, 23, 27, 31-33, 37-39, 41, 58, 59, 72, 91, 101, 102, 128
Ionizing radiation 46
Iron 46, 97, 105, 129, 132
Iron deficiency 22, 159
Irradiation 46, 103, 105, 124
Irritability 33, 36, 41, 96, 117, 139, 157, 162
Irritable bowel syndrome 15, 31, 41, 53, 65, 107, 117, 127, 146, 147, 154

J

Jaundice 60-62
Jawbone cavitation 47
Jejunum 7
Jock itch 32
Joint 14, 33, 40, 75, 106
    aches 85
    pain 36, 90, 159
Juice 23, 87, 88
    diet 86-88, 130
    recipes 87
Juicing 87, 97, 106, 111, 113

K

Kefir 100, 105
Kelp 50, 117, 134
Kidney 45, 46, 49, 50, 81, 130
    stones 139, 147

L

L-glutamine 9, 73, 96, 107, 108, 151, 164
L-leucine 118
Lactic acid 103, 104, 143
Lactis 100
Lacto-vegetarian 132
Lactobacillus 10, 99-103, 105, 164

acidophilus 10, 99, 100, 102, 103, 105, 134, 145, 150, 153, 164
bifidus 103, 150, 153
brevis 100
bulgaricus 100, 101
casei 99-101
delbrueckii 100
faecalis 100
faecium 100, 102
infantis 100, 104, 105, 164
kefir 100, 105
lactis 100
longum 100, 104
plantarum 100
salivarius 100, 103
yoghurti 100
Bifidus 103, 150, 153
Brevis 100
Bulgaricus 100, 101
Casei 99-101
Delbrueckii 100
Faecalis 100
Faecium 100, 102
Infantis 100, 104, 105, 164
Kefir 100, 105
Lactis 100
Longum 100, 104
Plantarum 100
Salivarius 100, 103
Yoghurti 100
Lactose 103, 144, 145, 147
    intolerance 39, 144, 146, 147
Large intestine 3, 8-10, 38, 39, 84, 86, 100, 101, 103, 104, 139, 146
Laxatives 45, 85, 129
Lead 46, 49, 52, 159
Leaky gut syndrome 27, 32, 38, 40-, 41, 46, 55, 139
Learning disability 159, 160
Lemon 97, 133
    grass 95
    juice 88, 94, 115, 135
Lifestyle 37, 38, 69, 77, 121, 123, 130, 141
Ligaments 60
Liver 3, 6-8, 12-14, 26, 27, 29, 32-33, 36, 41, 43, 45, 46, 49, 50, 53, 55-64, 68, 75, 77, 79-81, 93, 103, 106, 111, 113-115, 118, 124, 137, 139, 144, 148, 154
    cancer 46, 62
    detox 59
    detoxification 89, 111-114
    disease 46, 55, 61
    distress 117
    dysfunction 55, 60, 61
    enzyme 113
    herbal detox 113
    impairment 56
    spots 117
    test 118
    toxicity 114
Lo han 78, 94, 95, 135, 158, 162
Longum 100, 104
Low fat diet 124

Acknowledgment
Technical illustrations provided by
Dorling Kindersley© London, England